Breast cancer: Sharing the decision

Edited by

ANNA M. MASLIN

International Nursing Officer, the Department of Health, England
Visiting Professor, Faculty of Health,
Social work and Education,
University of Northumbria at Newcastle

Formerly

Senior Clinical Nurse Specialist—Breast Group Unit Manager
The Royal Marsden NHS Trust—Institute of Cancer Research
London and Sutton

With

TREVOR J. POWLES

Consultant Medical Oncologist
Head of the Breast Group
The Royal Marsden NHS Trust—Institute of Cancer Research
London and Sutton

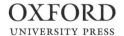

OXFORD
UNIVERSITY PRESS

OXFORD
UNIVERSITY PRESS

Great Clarendon Street, Oxford OX2 6DP

Oxford University Press is a department of the University of Oxford
and furthers the University's aim of excellence in research, scholarship,
and education by publishing worldwide in
Oxford New York

Athens Auckland Bangkok Bogota Buenos Aires Calcutta
Cape Town Chennai Dar es Salaam Delhi Florence Hong Kong Istanbul
Karachi Kuala Lumpur Madrid Melbourne Mexico City Mumbai
Nairobi Paris São Paulo Singapore Taipei Tokyo Toronto Warsaw
and associated companies in
Berlin Ibadan

Oxford is a registered trade mark of Oxford University Press

Published in the United States
by Oxford University Press, Inc., New York

© A.M. Maslin and the contributors listed on p. ix, 1999

The moral rights of the author have been asserted

First published 1999

British Library Cataloguing in Publication Data

Library of Congress Cataloging in Publication Data

1 3 5 7 9 10 8 6 4 2

ISBN 0 19 262967 0

Typeset by Newgen Imaging Systems (P) Ltd, Chennai, India
Printed in Great Britain on acid free paper by
Biddles Ltd., Guildford, Surrey

Contents

Contents

The views expressed in this book are those of the authors and are not a statement of Government Policy

Acknowledgements

The Royal Marsden NHS Trust and Institute for Cancer Research
The King's Fund Centre for Development, London
The BUPA Medical Foundation
Breast Cancer Care
CancerBACUP
Cancerlink
The Irish Cancer Society
Macmillan Cancer Relief
TAK TENT—Cancer Support Scotland
Tenovus Cancer Information Centre
The Ulster Cancer Foundation
The Patients, their families and friends without whom this work
    would not have been possible.
also
Mrs Wendy Cooper
Mrs Geraldine Doyle
Dr Andree' Le May
Mrs Kate Nash
Mr Andrew Prouse
Ms Helen Rowlands
Mrs Jane Walters
Mrs Beverly Akwara
Stephen, Sarah, Alex and Charlotte

Contributors

Mrs A. Ardern-Jones, The Institute of Cancer Research, Cancer Genetics Unit, 15 Cotswold Road, Sutton, Surrey, UK.

Dr Laura Assersohn, The Royal Marsden NHS Trust Breast Unit, Sutton, Surrey SM2 5PT

Dr Angela Coulter, Executive Director, Policy and Development, The Kings Fund 11–13 Cavendish Square, London, W1M 0AN

Dr Rosalind Eeles, Clinical Senior Lecturer & Honorary Consultant in Cancer Genetics & Clinical Oncology, The Institute of Cancer Research & Royal Marsden NHS Trust, Cancer Genetics Team, 15 Cotswold Road, Sutton Surrey, SM2 5NG, UK.

Dr Rosalind Given-Wilson, Consultant Radiologist, South West London Breast Screening Service, The Duchess of Kent Unit, London SW17 0BZ

Dr Tim Habeshaw, Consultant Clinical Oncologist, The Beatson Oncology Centre, Western Infirmary, Glasgow

Professor Anna Maslin, International Nursing Officer, the Dept. of Health, England formerly, Senior Clinical Nurse Specialist—Breast Group Unit Manager, The Royal Marsden NHS Trust—Institute of Cancer Research, London

Ms Gaye McPhail—Macmillan Lecturer, Practitioner in Cancer Nursing, Nursing and Midwifery School, University of Glasgow, 68 Oakfield Ave Glasgow G12 8LS

Dr Trevor Powles, Consultant Medical Oncologist, Head of the Breast Group, The Royal Marsden NHS Trust—Institute of Cancer Research

Mr Anthony Skene, Consultant Breast Surgeon, The Breast Unit, The Royal Bournemouth Hospital, Bournemouth BH7 7DW

Dr I.E. Smith, Head of Section of Medicine, The Royal Marsden NHS Trust, Fulham Rd. London SW3 6JJ

Mrs Jan Secker Walker, Research Sister, Action against Breast Cancer University College London Medical School, Department of Surgery, London W1P 7LD formerly, Honorary Clinical Nurse Specialist, The Royal Marsden Hospital NHS Trust, London

Preface

Breast cancer, decisions and dilemmas

Great debate surrounds the issue of patients with breast cancer participating in surgical/medical decision-making and their ability to give an informed consent (Baum 1982; Baum and Houghton 1988; Tobias 1992; Williams 1992; Maslin 1994). Health care professionals must balance the need to safeguard the rights of patients, respect their autonomy, and yet be sensitive to the changes and individual variations patients may demonstrate as they progress from diagnosis to the end point of their disease (Gillon 1992; Maslin 1994).

Providing information is only one part of the process of enabling patients to share more fully in decisions about their care if they so wish. Making information meaningful and the choices realistic means addressing how health care is being delivered and making appropriate changes as necessary. Questions arise relating to who should provide the information and how the information given to patients can be made consistent and unambiguous. What is the effect of consultant staff, junior doctors and different grades of nursing staff all giving information to patients? If information about choices is given to patients, does the health care setting allow patients to exercise choice? If not, is the result increased frustration for patients? Are patients more satisfied with the care they receive if they are informed and share the decision-making process? These are questions which clinicians and patients increasingly debate.

The anxiety and depression found in women with early breast cancer can be reduced if they are seen by a clinician who communicates effectively with them and who aims to incorporate patient choice into treatment decisions when possible if the patient wishes. Women receiving treatment for breast cancer constitute a patient group in whom some, but not all, of the questions surrounding communication choice and shared decision-making have been explored (Maslin et al. 1998).

The framework underpinning this book is based on a discussion of the ethical principles combined with an appreciation of the known benefit to women with a diagnosis of breast cancer if they have information relating to their disease and treatment options communicated to them effectively. This is taken one step further if a woman is to be involved in decisions relating to her care. If a woman wishes to participate in treatment decisions she needs accurate, evidence-based, clinically effective information to enable her to make an informed choice when considering options for the treatment of the cancer in her breast. Fundamental to this is an awareness of the literature which explores medical ethics in relation to beneficence, maleficience, personal autonomy, informed consent and advocacy which impacts on the decisions whether to provide or deny a woman access to explicit information. Having accurate information means the ability to access up-to-date, evidence-based medicine (EBM), the quality of which has been evaluated, thus enabling the individual woman to exercise a choice, although as will be discussed, accessing information is usually not enough. The individual woman needs to know how the information relating to the disease and treatment options applies to her own case. At this time many women are emotionally vulnerable and often need a high level of psychological care accompanied by clear, empathetic communication within the breast cancer setting.

This book aims to address the issues relating to shared decision-making, in particular in those areas where a choice of treatment option involves some degree of risk/benefit analysis. Although books describing early breast cancer treatment options exist, few, if any, deal with the subject in this way, focusing on the real dilemma that faces both clinician and patient if they wish to form a partnership in the decision-making process. While general principles of treatment are known, decisions in breast cancer treatment are often relative, with clinicians weighing up potential benefit against potential harm to an individual's length and/or quality of life. If life or cure could be guaranteed these decisions would not present such a dilemma.

At the time of diagnosis a woman is vulnerable. She has entered a world in which she perceives her life to be at risk and where she may not already possess the basic information on which to base any treatment decision, should she wish to make one. In the past if a woman was told a mastectomy would save her life she was very rarely in a position to argue the relative merits of one treatment over another, even if she knew what they were. The situation today is often different, with clinicians frequently having to share their uncertainty and debate treatment merits.

This book focuses on the question of how decisions about treatments are faced rather than the treatments themselves. It is different in that patients and leading breast cancer experts have been asked to share some of their own personal experiences of handling difficult decisions.

We feel sure this book will be of benefit to anyone who is thinking through, or working with, the day-to-day reality of breast cancer treatment decisions.

Newcastle A.M.M.
November 1998

Introduction

A. Maslin and T.J. Powles

Breast cancer is a chronic and unpredictable disease (Powles and Smith 1991). Approximately 25 000–26 000 women are diagnosed with cancer of the breast every year in the UK and approximately 15 000–16 000 die of the disease annually (Rubens 1992; Cancer Research Campaign 1996). Research effort has been aimed at trying to identify high-risk women, to prevent the disease (Powles and Smith 1991), to cure early primary breast cancer (Early Breast Cancer Trialists' Collaborative Group 1992; Rubens 1992; Sacks and Baum 1993; British Association of Surgical Oncology (BASO) 1994; British Breast Group (BBG) 1995) and to address the issues surrounding locally advanced/metastatic cancer of the breast (Powles and Smith 1991). While general principles of treatment are known (Powles and Smith 1991; Sacks and Baum 1993; British Association of Surgical Oncology 1994; British Breast Group 1995; Baum and Saunders 1994), decisions in breast cancer treatment are often relative, with clinicians weighing up the potential benefits against any potential harm to an individual's length and/or quality of life. If additional years of life or cure could be guaranteed these decisions would not present such a dilemma for the clinician or the patient.

Breast cancer assaults a woman on a number of different levels: there is the physical, psychological, emotional, and spiritual (Maguire *et al.* 1980; 1988*a,b,c*; Baum and Saunders 1994). Physically, the woman is facing diagnostic tests, the possibility of surgery—whether a wide local excision or mastectomy ± reconstruction, the possibility of radiotherapy, the possibility of systemic therapy and, if premenopausal, the possibility of her fertility being affected (Fallowfield and Clark 1991; Baum and Saunders 1994). Psychologically, she is coping with the possibility of a threat to her life, the possibility of a change to her life goals, and in some cases fairly severe anxiety and or depression.

Maguire *et al.* (1978, 1980) established that there is a known psychiatric morbidity 1 : 4 among women who have faced a diagnosis of breast cancer. Emotionally, a woman may experience mood fluctuation due to the general situation but also for some women the situation is aggravated by an early menopause induced by systemic treatment and/or ovarian oblation (Powles and Smith 1991). Spiritually, women are challenged either in their belief or non-belief in an afterlife, in their attitudes and values to this life, and in their approach to the coming months and years (Kifr and Slevin 1991).

At the time of a breast cancer diagnosis a woman is vulnerable. She has entered a world in which she perceives her life to be at risk and where she may not already possess the basic information on which to base any treatment decision should she wish to make one. In the past if a woman was told a mastectomy would save her life she was very rarely in a position to argue the relative merits of one treatment over another even if she knew what they were.

The theoretical framework underpinning this book is based on the premise that there are ethical principles which call for the respect of an individual's expression of personal autonomy and self determination in the normal course of events (Harris 1985; Glover 1990; Gillon 1992). This is combined with an appreciation of the known benefit to women with a diagnosis of breast cancer, if they desire it, of having information relating to their disease and treatment options communicated to them effectively (Fallowfield *et al.* 1990*a,b*; Mort 1996). This thinking is taken one step further when a woman wishes to express her autonomy and be involved in decisions relating to her care. If this is a course of action she wishes to opt for she needs accurate, evidence-based, clinically effective information to enable her to make an informed choice when considering options for the treatment of the cancer in her breast (Hack *et al.* 1994; Mort *et al.* 1995; NHS Executive Clinical Outcomes Group 1996). Underpinning this thinking is an awareness of the wider literature which explores medical ethics in relation to beneficence, maleficience, informed consent, and advocacy which impacts on the decisions whether to provide or deny a woman access to explicit information. Having accurate information requires the ability to access up-to-date, evidence-based medicine (EBM), the quality of which has been evaluated, thus enabling the individual woman to exercise a choice (Dixon 1996; Mort 1996), although accessing information is usually not enough. The individual woman needs to know how the information relating to the disease and treatment options applies to her own case. This is important as we know at the time of diagnosis many women are emotionally vulnerable and often need a high level of psychological care accompanied by clear empathetic communication within the breast cancer setting (Maguire *et al.* 1980; Watson *et al.* 1988.).

The literature review in this book has focused on five key areas

1. The ethical issues that have an effect on a patient's ability to access treatment-related information including the impact of deontology, utilitarianism, respect for autonomy, the role of informed consent, and advocacy.

2. The impact of the move towards evidence-based medicine on women now facing treatment choices.

3. The role of communication in the effort to access information and the impact of psychiatric morbidity on a breast cancer patient's ability to benefit from this information.

4. The practicalities of accessing good-quality information and the relationship between accessing information and decision-making.

5. A survey of the approaches to shared decision-making and a brief evaluation of their role, including the role of computerized interactive videos.

1

Sharing the dilemma

Anna M. Maslin

The patient's dilemma

To set the scene for this book, here is the true account of one patient's journey through her diagnosis, decision-making process, and treatment for breast cancer. It is her story and unique to her. It does not represent the experiences of all women and yet there are themes which recur in many accounts. This patient was chosen at random, not because her story was a 'good' experience or a 'bad' experience. As professionals we often only see in part what the patient experiences as a whole. On occasions it is sometimes helpful to see the situation from the patient's point of view.

Jane

Although my story may seem a series of catastrophes, the experience proved to be a positive one. I went from being a passive, accepting person to one who now feels much more in control and more positive. In 1981, our son went to prep school aged nine. Unfortunately he was unhappy there. It was a very traumatic and emotional time for us as a family. We told him at half-term that he was going to leave the school but we all suffered for half a term while he was still there. It seemed like an eternity and during that time I began to feel quite breathless. Looking back I think it was just sheer angst. I went to the doctor because I thought perhaps I had a heart condition or something.

The doctor examined my breasts and said he had found a lump. It was about the size of a little dry pea. This was the autumn term and he suggested I came back before Christmas just to see if it had altered. By Christmas it hadn't changed in shape or size. I was quite happy with it and so was he so we did nothing about it. I was 37 years old at the time. I suppose I was quite young and so we felt confident it wasn't anything serious and left it. Within quite a short period of time I virtually forgot about it.

About five years later in 1986 I thought I'd better have an 'MOT' and so went for a private well woman check-up. At the check-up they noticed the lump and so I had a mammogram. The mammogram showed up little calcifications. As a result things began to happen fairly quickly and my own family doctor referred me to a specialist cancer centre. He was very supportive.

I had a lumpectomy in June 1986 and was diagnosed with *in situ* breast cancer. To tell the truth I didn't really think too much about it. It was very painful but I recovered well and after two years I just let it go. I had lots of check-ups and my final mammogram was in May 1993. It was nearing 10 years by then and all seemed clear.

I had my fiftieth birthday in November 1993 which was fantastic. I was on top of the world although I felt quite tired. A week later I was rushing around early in the morning because of the busy day ahead, but I was conscious of having insistent little pains in my breast that I'd been ignoring as I'd been too busy. In the bathroom I popped my hand on my breast and felt a lump. This lump was different from the first one—it was like a knuckle. I felt it through my nightdress. I said to David, my husband, 'Oh God, I've got a lump'. I booked myself straight in to see my consultant.

I saw the consultant the following week. I wasn't overly worried because the Breast Unit had been keeping such a good eye on me and because I had had the experience of *in situ* cancer and this lump was in exactly the same place. When I went up to the hospital I actually took a packed hold-all with me because I thought they'd whisk me straight in. But no—I had a late appointment. It was a long time before I was seen so it was just before everything closed. The consultant confirmed he could feel a lump but said 'I think it's probably going to be hormonal. Don't worry about it, come back in a month and we'll see how it goes'. Because I had my period and everything I accepted this, but when I was getting dressed I was suddenly overcome with this feeling: this is not right, did he feel what I felt? It was so obvious to me what it was that when I got dressed I called a nurse and said 'I really need to talk to the consultant again because I'm really not happy'.

The nurse relayed messages and in the end the consultant came out and spoke to me. I explained I really was unhappy about this lump and I just didn't feel that I wanted to wait for a month. I didn't feel it was hormonal. I felt it was something serious. The consultant listened and said 'If it is cancer I can absolutely guarantee it will be *in situ* cancer, so don't worry about it'. I saw him on 23 November and as my next appointment was for 7 December I decided to wait that time to see whether it was hormonal or not. I felt very reassured by him being so definite.

I went back on 7 December and they drew off some liquid from the lump. Once again I had a late appointment so I couldn't have a mammogram because the department was shut. The nursing staff were very good and said that next time I would be given a form to enable me to have the mammogram first, prior to the appointment. On 14 December I got the results and was told there was something amiss, and so I had a core biopsy which I think was clear. There was some contradiction here and so I had another appointment and my case was discussed with a professor. They thought, in view of my history, I ought to have a biopsy, although they were even at that time quite sure that it would be *in situ cancer*. By then I was sure there was something amiss but because I'd had it before I wasn't bothered really. I went on a very nice holiday and my biopsy was scheduled for 5 January.

The day before the operation I stayed the night in London and went to the hospital the following day as a day patient. I was given all the usual checks before I went down to surgery. There was a backlog so I was on the trolley for a long time but that didn't bother me. While I was on the trolley, just about to go in to the theatre, the professor came past and the person who was going to do the operation—I never did discover who it was—said to him 'I'd like you to check this patient'. So I was sitting on the trolley with my notes on my knee and the professor was sheafing through and said 'In view of her history, I just have a hunch. I think you should go for it'. I asked 'What does that mean?' and he said I should have a wide local excision rather than a simple biopsy. I wasn't worried by this, in fact it felt good to be a part of the decision-making process. I appreciated the fact it was happening there in front of me. Other people might think how awful—having your notes on your knee—but I liked that. I preferred to be involved. Shortly after that I went in and had it done but I was surprised at how much was taken away. It seemed like a piece of breast tissue the size of my hand was removed, leaving quite a big scar.

When I came round I went back into the day ward. The events that followed felt like a nightmare. I realized that I couldn't take morphine because I hallucinate terribly. My blood pressure was very low. I lay there recovering but I felt very dizzy, sick, and I was in a great deal of pain. I had a suppository for the sickness and pain. At about four o'clock they came and sat me up but I was feeling dreadful. The 'powers that be' came round and said they didn't have a bed for me to stay overnight. I felt that I had to get myself together enough to get home because they kept coming to check on me and saying 'Well, I don't know. Perhaps you will be okay to get home'.

David came at five o'clock. It was decided that I was well enough to go home and he had to dress me. It was just dreadful. At that time I was the sort of person that wanted to please, wanted to be okay, to fit in. I wasn't well enough to go home and I knew that. Feeling very sick I managed to get to the car. It was a two and a half hour drive home. I was constantly being sick into some bags I'd been given. I hadn't been round from the anaesthetic very long and my scar was painful—it was about four and a half inches long. I also had awful diarrhoea from the suppository. I was having to stop at service stations, looking like death, rolling into the lavatories and coming out again. I mean, it was just horrific. I finally got back home and thankfully got into bed. It was late at night and no home care had been arranged.

I was at home until I returned on 14 January to have my one continuous stitch removed. The pain had continued and quite a lot of fluid had collected in the wound. While I was waiting in the cubicle for the fluid to be drained off, a young chap stuck his head round the curtain and said 'Oh Mrs ***, we're going to have to do some more surgery'. Those were his first words to me before he'd even come in. David was sitting in the out-patients because neither of us were expecting any unusual news—simply that it was *in situ* breast cancer which we had coped with before.

So that was a huge shock. David was out there in the waiting room and I was in there on my own, and I had this news that it was whatever—I can't remember exactly what he said—but it was not *in situ*, it was invasive breast cancer and they wanted to have a look to see if it had spread. I remember looking at the nurse who was very sweet and supportive but it was like I'd actually gone into shock so I kept thinking 'Well, I've just got to cope with this'. It didn't occur to me to say 'David's out there—can he come in?'

My initial reaction was that I couldn't stand any more surgery just then because it was only, what, nine days since the last operation? I told them I couldn't bear the thought of any more surgery. I kept saying over and over 'I just can't!' They said 'Well, we'll make a date. It doesn't matter for a few weeks but we would like to do it fairly quickly'. Looking back, at that point I should have been asked by someone if I had anyone with me. How was I going to get home? What was my situation?

To complicate matters the operation diary had gone AWOL so we couldn't sort out the date. At that point I came out of the examination room and went over to David. I think he saw the look on my face. We were both in shock. Because of the situation with the diary I then had to make my own appointment. For some reason it was very difficult to get through to the secretary. I did manage it in the end and we made an appointment for me to come into hospital to have the operation but this would be confirmed. I didn't hear anything from the hospital so after a while I did check up to see why I hadn't received confirmation. It was quite extraordinary. When I rang I was told that my bed had gone. I lost my slot because somebody who was more needy had taken it. They hadn't let me know, so we had to make another appointment for me to come in.

I finally came in on 27 January and saw a really nice young doctor who was sort of preparing me. He did an examination of my breasts prior to the operation the next day. At that time I was very stiff, I couldn't get my arm up. I think I had so much scar tissue in the breast that the scar had shrivelled and my breast was all puckered up and pointing upwards. It looked a real mess. I felt it was horrible. The doctor bent over and said to me 'Oh you have been unlucky here'. As a result we got talking about possible treatments and I suddenly had this idea. I think I said 'Oh well, I might as well have the whole lot taken away, it looks so awful'. I then asked 'If I have a mastectomy, will I have to have radiotherapy?'. The doctor replied 'No, you won't'. So that set me thinking.

The following day I had my axilla operation. I know this sounds like one long moan, but I didn't have a very good experience coming round from that operation because there were two people in recovery, a man and a woman, who were talking endlessly about the theatre, everything and anything, but not to me. Finally someone else came over and took charge—she was absolutely super. I came back to the ward and recovered well. It was a Wednesday I think, but by the weekend I knew that I really wanted to talk about having a mastectomy and what that would involve.

I got an appointment to see the surgeon who had done the operation but was somewhat saddened at his reaction which was what a pity it was I hadn't made up my mind before, because they could have saved on the surgery time and bed space and I could have had the whole lot done on the Thursday. I explained that I hadn't had the idea until the Wednesday and it was really rather close to have made such a major decision. I think he was very pressured. I could understand his position but I found it was the last straw. After he'd gone I burst into tears and the staff all rushed around. It was then I knew I needed to take control and it was then that I decided I wanted to know everything about what having a mastectomy would entail.

For whatever reason it was only at that point that I met the breast care nurse who was great. For the first time I began to access more detailed information. I really felt that I was being heard and began to get the kind of information and psychological support I needed. Another thing that happened was because I was so distressed they sent me a young man—I don't know who he was. He came and sat with me for half an hour and I was able to tell him my story about the day surgery and all the things that had gone wrong. I told him how I really felt and he wrote it all down in my notes. I really felt a lot better because it had been a series of misses somehow. I'd coped with each one and made allowances each time, and then reached the final straw.

On 4 February I came back for the results of my axillary surgery and received good news—the axilla was clear. So for me the prospect of any further chemotherapy treatment seemed to be fading. David and I were so happy we thought we'd go down to the pub and have some champagne. We didn't actually get there because I was also given the news that because of the nature of the cancer, they did want to give me chemotherapy. This was obviously another shock but this time I was being told in a more caring way. David was with me. I felt I had options, I felt I could be part of the decision-making process. It was presented very well—I was informed this is what they would like me to do, I didn't have to, but they recommended it. There was no problem except that more chemotherapy was the one thing that I had really dreaded.

Once I came home I rang Cancer BACUP and a friend who was a breast surgeon in Leeds who was absolutely brilliant. She gave me endless time, hours and hours, talking through on the telephone the mastectomy, the possibility of reconstruction, chemotherapy, radiotherapy, and all I wanted to know. I really felt I wanted to make a decision for myself, with guidance obviously, but I felt it needed to be an informed decision. I read lots of material from a variety of sources.

When I saw the surgeon next time I said that I had decided I would like to have a mastectomy and he suggested that I saw the professor again to talk it all through. I think this time they could sense that I was really serious and that I really needed to go to the top. The surgeon suggested if I had a mastectomy I might want to consider an immediate reconstruction, but I had decided I didn't want a reconstruction at that point. I felt if I was unhappy with the mastectomy after, say, six months, I could perhaps have an implant then. The surgeon wasn't too happy. He said he would prefer to do the reconstruction at the same time and take it out if I was unhappy with the result. I knew I didn't want to do it that way round. I felt I could cope with a mastectomy but I wasn't sure. I felt like I was on the top diving board looking down in to the swimming pool way beneath, about to jump and not knowing how I'd land, or how I'd feel when I landed. I thought I'd be all right but I really didn't know.

When I did see the professor he said that if the cancer recurred then they would definitely give me a mastectomy, but I thought 'I'm not waiting for that'. I'd had enough. I had carefully considered all the possibilities. As the professor spoke to me I looked him in the eye and said 'Would you do this operation for me?', and he agreed. He informed me that the statistics for a lumpectomy, chemotherapy, and radiotherapy were as good as mastectomy and chemotherapy. I knew I had a choice and I felt happy that it was my choice. We booked in, and on 23 February I had the mastectomy.

Strangely enough from then on I felt good about everything that happened. I felt I was being consulted, I felt I was in control.

I had personal counselling which was brilliant. We had some really wonderful sessions about chemotherapy because I was very frightened about having it. It seemed to me that being sick was the only thing that seemed to stop me in my tracks. I hated feeling sick. It was a big thing for me to accept chemotherapy but I felt I needed to give myself and my family every opportunity for me to remain well. I wanted us all to know that I had done all I could, so that if I had died there wouldn't have been a question mark for them of 'if only she'd had the chemotherapy'.

For me, once the chemotherapy was completed that was the end of all my treatment. I had the mastectomy prior to the chemotherapy and I had the most beautiful scar compared to the first one. After the operation I had the physiotherapy provided by the hospital but I was also able to arrange some locally as I felt that once a week was not going to be enough. My local physiotherapist massaged my scar. She gave me the confidence that I could stretch and not do any damage. She tailored a programme of exercises for me to do. I took it all very seriously, spending at least half an hour a day, and that paid off well. I was worried about possible scar tissue building up underneath—I didn't want a repeat of my first experience. We really took care of the scar and I'm so pleased with the result.

When I saw the professor in the out-patients department he made a comment about my attitude to the operation which was so valuable to me.

When I had the lumpectomy, the first time I saw the scar was when I took the dressing off at home. I nearly fainted because it was such a shock to see the scar which seemed so long. I was so upset I felt cold and clammy and had to go to bed. After the mastectomy, I had a transparent dressing on my scar so I was able to look down and see it straight away. I know that wouldn't suit some people but for me it was brilliant because there was nothing hidden. There was nothing I had to steel myself to see. Another important aspect for me was that when I came round from the operation I could take the bed covers off to look down at the flat chest on that side. It wasn't a shock because I remembered pre-puberty. Odd as it may seem, I felt I'd only gone back in time. For me it wasn't like losing a limb that you've always had, it was quite different and it really helped me a lot to realize that.

I never did have a reconstruction. The breast care nurse arranged for me to meet someone on the ward who'd had a reconstruction and have a look. The reconstructed breast looked very good but I still thought that if I could go it alone without any other complications I would be happier. I preferred the simplicity and so far I am absolutely satisfied with it.

The experience of having my prosthesis fitted was good. My daughter came with me and she said 'Yes mum, that looks all right'. For me there was no problem at all. It was all done in a caring but matter-of-fact way.

I don't know why but the mastectomy was very painful because of the nature of the operation and the stretching of the skin to meet the old scar, but the scar itself never bothered me. When I came home a week after I'd had the operation, the first night I was at home with David, who was in bed, I just stripped off as I normally do and turned towards him to get my nightdress out of the bed, not even thinking about it. He didn't make it an issue—I knew he was totally accepting and I somehow accepted it too. I think it was because I had done all the work previously and it wasn't imposed.

Prior to the mastectomy I came across a useful psychological exercise in a magazine. What it suggested was that, if you were going to lose a part of yourself, to work through the grieving process in advance. So that's what I did with my counsellor. I used to visualize my breast before it came away. I would visualize letting go of it, and saying goodbye to it, and really appreciating its usefulness, and all the rest of it, then letting it go. After that, for me the operation was a doddle. I can't really explain it. I was completely without worry, without fear, without embarrassment, without self-consciousness. It was quite extraordinary.

The partner's dilemma

David

When Jane was diagnosed with invasive breast cancer it was in many ways like picking up a thread because of her previous experience. In a sense it was like rediscovering where we were before and then going forward with it. The immediate fear that everybody has, I think, and it was in my case, in both our cases, is how we would view the continuity of life. There is the theoretical abstract reasoning but individually, personally, of course, there's the immediate personal fear of 'I'm going to be alone'. I suppose most people would share that fear. Jane and I share a philosophy of life which has helped us face the prospect of death, but nevertheless, personal fears and hopes remain, so there is a real contradiction. It's not black or white, it's sort of feeling both things at the same time.

Jane was at first concerned primarily with survival and then later she took a more philosophical perspective. For me, being immediately faced with the possibility of Jane's non-survival you wonder how it will be, how it will be for Jane, how it will be for me. You wonder, how will I cope, can I cope with the process, can I cope with the possible loss? That's the sort of wondering— will I rise to our ideals—knowing that, theoretically, yes I could but wondering whether, in fact, I could.

In relation to taking part in decisions, with Jane, on occasions I was not physically present to support her. This was not through any fault of our own but because of the circumstances; for example, when she was on the trolley just prior to theatre or when she initially received the diagnosis of invasive cancer. Having said that, however, I felt very much that Jane was the one who basically needed to decide. I didn't ever feel that somehow I needed to make the decisions for her. I didn't feel very well equipped to make decisions for her anyway. I never felt that it was down to me to make the decision, to take it away from her, because she was both emotionally and mentally able to grapple with it herself. I saw my role as supporting Jane in whatever course of action she felt was right.

I wanted to participate in the decision-making process by being there for Jane and on occasions giving my view but not in terms of feeling she must do this or she should do that. I thought very much that she intuitively sensed the right thing to do. I was happy to support Jane in this way because I felt my view was by definition mine and therefore slightly biased, which it had to be in some senses.

One thing I did feel is that we could have had loads, loads, loads more information both at the beginning and also through the course of events. The outside help that we had was tremendous, but it wasn't through the system—it was through BACUP and through a friend who was a breast surgeon. Gathering information wasn't a coping strategy in itself for me. I didn't think that activity was the solution, but without adequate information you can't make a reasoned decision. In terms of seeking out the information it was very much Jane who was doing the searching and I was there as a support. She was the one who actually did the pursuing and my impression is that the information wasn't easily available.

As the husband I felt I was not given the information that would have been helpful, not just in terms of anatomy or treatments but also in terms of support. As it was, Jane felt able to pursue her information needs and she was able to take control. If Jane had been a different person, someone who was unable or unwilling to access what she needed, then that might have forced me to take a more proactive role. I felt that if she needed me to then I would have had to become involved, although I expect I would have found it quite difficult.

There seems to be a combination of factors which makes accessing information difficult. Hospitals and doctors are obviously busy people but there is also this culture of being busy, if you understand what I mean. The view seems to be the busier you are the more important you are. Oddly, on the whole, it doesn't apply to the nurses. Nurses were very good indeed. They had the time but were not always in the position to have all the information or take the decisions. In my view I think that probably there needs to be someone who has the time and expertise to answer the clinical questions, someone to provide the emotional support, and someone to answer the day-to-day queries. The whole information issue seems to get jumbled up as one. Questions on hospital visiting times are not questions the clinician wants to spend time answering, but there needs to be someone set aside who can answer these sort of disparate problems and then the clinician can concentrate on key issues like the prognosis which you really need to have answered but they never seem to have the time to address.

Sometimes key appointments with the consultant only lasted five minutes. Our consultation when Jane discussed the mastectomy with the professor was longer, although admittedly a lot of that time was in deciding whether he could find the time in his diary to do the operation. The hard-core discussions on the kind of issues like prognosis, options, risk, probability of success, and so on were very, very brief. There was a lot of time spent doing other things rather than actually giving the information or the answers to questions. In our case we had filled these information gaps from outside sources, but this is not always possible. Another issue professionals should take on board is the effort and time it often takes patients to get up to hospital, especially if they have travelled a long way. To wait for prolonged periods and spend often a very short period of time with the doctor is not really acceptable.

At the key appointments I would have preferred a clearer explanation of options rather than saying 'We recommend this' and leaving the patient to then come back with questions like 'Well what about so and so, and what if so and so', which in that style of interview situation you can't think of. You often only think about the key questions afterwards. If professionals were more analytical in their presentation, for example more willing to say 'These are the options: a, b, or c. With a the implications are i, ii, & iii but with b it is iv, v, & vi etc., and you also need to consider x, y, & z'—it would be much clearer. Often it seemed to me they were shooting from the hip. They may have been analysing the information themselves but I don't think they were thinking about presenting it logically. They would give a recommendation, a view, and that was it, not a multiple view. I suspect this way of working is not deliberate. It's subconscious. As it stands, based on the information we received at the hospital, without the additional information we accessed, we were not given adequate information on which to actually make a reasoned decision.

Another difficulty in the area of decision-making is that if you do have reasonably full information you may choose an option which is not the doctors' preferred choice. Our experience is that some doctors are not genuinely open to free choice in areas where a legitimate choice could be made. I think they would much rather you do what they recommend. I mean, in the case of reconstruction, for example, the whole idea that you should not have reconstruction is considered extraordinary. Why? Jane, for valid reasons, did not wish to have a reconstruction. They found this hard to accept. What was the basis for this fixed position? There was never any reason given for it. There wasn't 'Look, this is the situation—you can do this or you can do that'. It felt at times that if you went against their guidance, in a sense they were taking it a bit personally. It seemed to me they felt it was like a personal affront to their professional judgement. Their professional judgement is this and if you choose that, well, you know, you are rejecting their advice.

In my view, in areas where there is genuine choice, where there isn't an absolute right or wrong answer, if you are the sort of person that wants to be involved in the choice then you need to have that information.

Jane and David's adult son

All the information I had about my mother's breast cancer was relayed to me through my family, mainly through Jane and that tended to be based on what was happening at the time. In other words, she had got to a certain point and then I was told this was what was happening next. Jane shared her thoughts with me, for example that she had decided to do this or that, and my response was reactive to the situation rather than seeing how any of the decisions were made.

The year prior to Jane being diagnosed, a very good friend of mine's mother was diagnosed with breast cancer. She had had to take an active role but that was more because she had to convince her GP she had a lump, she was sure it was cancer, and she needed treatment. Jane's experience was dealt with in a totally different way. Sadly, my friend's mother is now dying. Overall, for me, it was a more positive experience because I saw it as more to do with getting well, although it was quite traumatic at the time. I even gave up smoking which pleased Jane. I only went up to the hospital once and that was enough. I felt quite distant and more reactive.

Jane seemed to have everything under control and my parents would update me as necessary. I never felt the need to actively seek any information. At the time, it seemed right. Looking back, however, it's always better to understand what someone is going through, so yes, in retrospect, to have been more involved and more fully informed may have been better because my view was based on this one view in my head which related to my friend and his mother.

On the whole I think I coped well. I guess I realized that Jane was finding out an awful lot of information. She was very well informed and therefore was able to answer my questions. She gave me the impression the situation was under control. I do have a sister but at the time she was abroad so I didn't have the opportunity to talk to her about the situation. I realize now Jane had some fairly traumatic experiences initially, but at first I wasn't totally aware of what was going on—but that is partly the way Jane is. She doesn't want to worry anyone so she won't tell anyone what's happening until she has an idea of the outcome—so you aren't overly involved. I didn't really understand exactly what the situation was until after the event and that sort of goes back to what I was saying to start with—it was more being updated on what was happening and what had happened than the dilemmas involved.

Postscript

Jane is keeping well, looking radiant, and her family remain a constant source of support to her.

2

Ethics and patient access to information

Anna M. Maslin

It may seem dry and uninspiring to look at the impact ethics has on a patient's ability to access information but the ethical position adopted by society and health care professionals can have a profound effect on a woman's ability to participate in treatment decision-making. Today in the West it would appear patients automatically have the right to health care information, but this may be a false premise. The premise that underpins the right of a patient, in this case a woman with breast cancer, to access information (or be protected from it if she wishes) is based on a number of ethical principles, e.g. beneficence (a duty to do her good), non-maleficence (a duty not to do harm), and respect for autonomy, to accord to the individual the full rights of self-determination (Glover 1990; Waldron 1990; Gillon 1992). There are two of the main moral theories: deontology and utilitarianism (Ross 1930; Kant 1964, 1973; Mill 1962a,b, 1974). These patient rights are interpreted differently depending on whether a deontological or utilitarian perspective are adopted (Kant 1964, 1973; Mill 1962a,b, 1974). Unless a case can be made for a woman having the right to access the information on which treatment decisions are made and which can impact on the quality and on occasions her quantity of her life, the issue of how a woman copes with different treatment options becomes immaterial. This section aims to review ethical principles which underpin a woman with breast cancer's right to access information or be protected from it.

Deontology

The term 'deontology' comes from the Greek word 'deon' meaning duty, not from the Latin 'deus' meaning God' (Gillon 1992).

It has come to represent the group of theories which are concerned with duty-based ethics. These theories focus in on the intrinsic rightness of an action (Kant 1964; 1973). The essence of morality depends on a person acting according to certain principles which are their duty (Ross 1930; Gillon 1992). This belief that a person simply by existing is owed certain rights (MacDonald 1990) can either come from a philosophical belief in a form of natural rights (Kant 1964; 1973; Geisler and Feinberg 1980) or it could be a directly prescribed belief from a religious conviction (Calvin 1960*a,b*; Tournier 1957; Cook 1983; Stout 1990). It could be argued health care professionals have a duty to tell patients the truth, if a duty to tell the truth generally exists in society (Kant 1964; 1973; Glover 1990; Waldron 1990; Gillon 1992).

MacDonald (1990) states:

'The word "right" has a variety of uses in ordinary language, which includes the distinction between "legal right" and "moral right". A has a legal right against B entails B has a duty to A which will be enforced by the courts. A has a claim against B recognized by an existing law. No person has a legal right which he cannot claim from some other (legal) person and which the law will not enforce. That A has a moral right against B likewise entails B has a duty to A. But it is not necessarily a duty which can be legally enforced. A has a right to be told the truth by B and B has a corresponding duty to tell A the truth. But no one, except in special circumstances recognized by law, can force B to tell the truth or penalize him except by censure if he does. No one can in general claim to be told the truth, by right, under penalty. But a creditor can claim repayment of a debt or sue his debtor.'

Telling the truth may cause harm, for instance psychological suffering, and therefore an alternative duty, the duty to do no harm, or non-maleficience, should take precedence (Tobias 1988). This can be seen for example in this illustration: if we cannot cure all cases of breast cancer, does a national breast screening programme help women by encouraging them to come for treatment earlier or does it simply give them more years to worry about the disease? Does the psychological harm in this case outweigh the benefit?

The classification of deontological theories

Deontological theories are concerned with types of action rather than with individual action (Kant 1964, 1973; cf. Beauchamp and Childress 1994).

Kantian philosophy/rule deontology

Immanuel Kant was a Prussian philosopher. Although he held Christian beliefs he was convinced a duty-based theory of rights could be hypothesized and defended independently of a faith in the existence of God or religious-based ethics. 'Kant believed that the truth of his moral theory was a necessary consequence of the rational nature of human beings. He believed that he could prove that any rational being necessarily recognized himself to be bound by what Kant called "the supreme moral law"' (Gillon 1992). This perspective suggested that consequences are not the issue when it comes to moral actions. All duties arrive from two universal principles (Kant 1964; 1973).

Kant expounded 'the principle of universality' that individuals must: (a) act as though your action could become a universal law applicable to all men; and (b) never treat yourself or another person as a means to an end. He developed a series of 'deontological precepts' which in summary included:

- to be moral a person must perform their preordained duty whatever the consequences
- some actions/obligations are right and good in themselves without regard to their consequences. They are not based on the ability to calculate consequences but on human reason. Because of this premise, philosophers have gone on to argue that generally it is right to save life rather than to kill (Glover 1990; Gillon 1992)
- although it is important to consider the consequences of action, some duties are supreme and have abiding importance, e.g. telling the truth or keeping promises. These duties are moral in themselves and just ought to be done by people. Although a woman may suffer by having the knowledge that she has a cancer diagnosis, it could be argued denying her the truth would cause greater harm.

Kant (1964) held that 'to duty every other motive must give place because duty is a condition of will good in itself, whose worth transcends everything' and that 'a truly moral act is not influenced by self-interest, nor by consideration of overall social benefit. The key to morality is that the person who is acting must do so out of pure motive of doing their moral duty'.

The 'Kantian categorical imperative' promoted the view that:

- act only on that maxim which you can at the same time will to be a universal law
- always treat human beings as ends in themselves and neither as a means to further ambitions and ends of others
- act as a member of a community where all the other members are 'ends' just as you are (Kant 1964; 1973).

These principles provide the basis of Kant's deontological theory which he believed allowed for equal respect for persons inspired by ideas of impartiality and forces a person to examine their conscience. The concept of 'ends' provides a standard by which to assess if an action is right or wrong. If mutual respect operates this should allow freedom in decision-making. On the other hand, it could be argued that it is impractical for certain duties to become universal laws.

How realistic is it not to take account of the consequences of actions? In the case of a woman with breast cancer it could be argued from this point of view that the woman may not have an intrinsic right to the truth because it may potentially cause her psychological harm through fear or worry. There is also a problem with the concept of 'ends'. There is often a conflict between theory and reality. Resources are not unlimited and therefore decisions are often made which consider more than the person as an end in themselves.

Failure to observe the precepts results in standards being bent or overruled, leading to a 'slippery slope' where responses are made contingently according to what seems to be right at the time (Beauchamp and Childress 1994). If basic duties are shunned, some individuals could rationalize immoral acts in pseudomoral language. For example, if a clinician finds it personally difficult to cope with the strong emotions a woman may express at the time of her diagnosis with breast cancer, he may choose not to tell a patient the full facts of her disease and he may rationalize this to himself by concluding it was not in her best interests to know such distressing information. Kant (1964; 1973) suggests even if it appears better to break faith in the short term, the consequences will not be better in the long term. 'Breaking faith' in this context would be the clinician making the decision not to tell the truth. The short-term benefit of the patient not knowing harmful information may result in her confusion when toxic or disfiguring treatments are suggested and/or her loss of trust in her clinician if she eventually discovers he withheld information from her.

Act deontology/a critical modification of utilitarianism

There are times when duties come into conflict, e.g. it may be right to tell the truth but if a terrorist asks me where my child is, I may refuse to tell the truth in order to save my child. Utilitarianism holds that the rightness of an action is based on the consequence of that action. There are duties in which there is a special relationship between the duty and the outcome. These duties are variable but often include duties of telling the truth, paying a debt, and being just. Scanlon (1990) stated deontologists 'frequently call attention to the abhorrent policies that unrestricted aggregate reasoning might justify under certain possible, or even actual, circumstances. They invite the conclusion that to do justice to the firm intuition that such horrors are clearly unjustified, one must adopt a deontological moral framework that places limits on what appeals to maximum aggregate well-being can justify'.

With this form of deontology:

- principles and duties for actions are not defined beforehand
- there is no onus to follow rigid rules
- the focus of moral action is not on rules but on informed human judgement in the context of each situation
- each situation is unique
- everything in morality rests upon the person who is to judge or decide
- the overriding duty in act deontology is for a person to be true to themselves (Ross 1930)

The advantages of this position are that a person is seen to be true to themselves, the uniqueness of each situation is acknowledged, and it claims to explode the myth of professional vs. personal conflict because the professional is duty bound to accord the person, i.e. the patient, their full rights. The disadvantages are that it can be impractical (could any health care system incorporate this theory?), it makes the assumption that everything about a given situation is unique, and who is to make the judgement about the duty owed in any particular situation?

For the woman with breast cancer this could mean that there is no general onus on the part of the health care professional to tell the truth to the patient and therefore the patient is left facing a situation in which the health care professional takes decisions and makes judgements based on their own assessment of each individual patient.

Merits of deontology

Deontological theory has an advantage in medical ethics. Actions as a result of this theory are predictable and standardized; therefore there should be a high code of clinical practice.

- Deontology seems closest to what could be described as ordinary daily ethics. In the Western world it is generally held that the truth must be told, people must not steal, justice is desirable, and autonomy should be respected. This reasoning would appear to support the view that rational patients should have their autonomy respected and therefore be given whatever information they request in order to enable them to make considered treatment choices (Gillon 1992; Maslin 1993; 1994; Baum 1994). This position does not exclude the possibility that some patients may choose to exercise their rights by delegating them to their clinician and this too is a valid treatment choice (Ingelfinger 1980; Fallowfield *et al.* 1990*a,b*; Maslin 1993; 1994; Baum 1994). There will also be for some an inability to express a rational treatment choice whether as a consequence of mental or physical impairment.
- Deontology acknowledges the diversity of moral relationships. Moral life is not seen just in terms of a means–end relationship, but as wealth of moral relationships, e.g. parent–child, husband–wife, employer–employee, or doctor–patient,

all which generate a different set of rights and duties (Ross 1930).

- Deontology acknowledges the importance of the past in generating moral duties. Duties can be owed because of promises or because of a previous relationship, e.g. he promised to marry her or the doctor promised to treat the patient.
- Deontology seems able to give the best account of justice which seems to underpin society.

Problems with deontology

- What happens when there is a conflict of moral duties? Which duty takes precedence: to tell the truth or to protect from psychological harm, e.g. to tell an asymptomatic woman she has metastatic breast cancer or to wait until she reports a problem? Ross (1930) distinguishes between prima facie rightness and actual rightness. An action is decided upon based on weighing up the situation. Some have developed 'lexical ordering' deontological duties. In this approach some rules or duties take precedence over others.
- Does deontology leave the individual with a plethora of confusing ultimate principles (Kerner 1990)? It could be suggested that the theory merely reflects the complexity of actual morality rather than trying to oversimplify reality. It is impossible to argue for absolute guidelines in truth telling for every individual. The Cancer Research Campaign Working Party (1983) accurately stated:

'To have a right is one matter. Choosing to exercise it is quite another. There will be some (perhaps many) who will decline to be fully informed but this pragmatic consideration cannot modify the intrinsic nature of the right itself. It is only the person who possesses the right, in this case the patient, who can decide whether she wishes to exercise it.'

- Does deontology result in the complete divorce of duty from action? If this is the case a person could in theory do his duty but cause considerable harm to others in the process. This is not in essence the case; a deontologist regards morality as a necessary part of a good life, not simply a means to it (Kant 1964; 1973).

Utilitarianism

Utilitarianism is a subset of consequentialism classically associated with the goal of happiness or pleasure (Sidgwick 1907; Bentham 1948; Mill 1871; 1962*a,b*; 1974). For consequentialists the rightness or wrongness of an act can only be judged on the grounds of whether its consequences (actual or intended) produce more benefits than disadvantages.

For utilitarians the essence of morality from this perspective rests upon a calculation of the benefits and disadvantages of the consequences of actions. Bentham's classical statement said 'A person should attempt to achieve the greatest happiness of the greatest number' (Bentham 1948). For Bentham the sole intrinsic good is pleasure and the sole intrinsic evil, pain. Other things are only bad or good in so far as they produce pain or pleasure (hedonism). The aim is to maximize (maximization) utilities like pleasure, happiness, and fulfilment there by minimizing negative quantities like pain, suffering, and misery.

The classification of utilitarian theories

Utilitarian theories are concerned with consequences of actions rather than with the duty owed to an action.

Basic utilitarianism

In this theory good, evil, happiness, and pleasure must be quantifiable. The decision-making agent must be considered of equal importance as others in the assessment of good, evil, etc. Agents must be impartial, disinterested, benevolent, and sacrifice self-interest to the general good (MacIntyre 1980; Singer 1994).

Act utilitarianism

In every situation an individual should assess which of the acts open to them is most likely to produce the greatest amount of good or evil, however defined (maximization), e.g. telling true but potentially upsetting information: one would be obliged to weigh up the pros and cons of telling the information in terms of the likely outcome—mental, physical, and social—to all concerned. Should women who carry a genetic predisposition to develop breast cancer be given this information? As the disease cannot for the present time be prevented, nor can all cases of breast cancer be guaranteed a cure (Powles and Smith 1991), this information is potentially harmful to the woman. She could be burdened with frightening information over which she has little control and which could affect her career prospects or eligibility to procure life insurance. The woman on the other hand may feel it is her right to know so she can exercise her autonomy by taking action to try and safeguard her health or decisions regarding her fertility and whether or not to have children who may also carry the gene(s).

Act utilitarianism can be seen as a form of opportunism in that it may allow evil actions to take place if the action produces more good than evil in the end. It may have the effect of diminishing professional integrity, e.g. if an antiemetic agent was in short supply and a wealthy person said they would fund more supplies provided they received treatment first, one could argue that the ends justify the means. The theory however is difficult in practice because we cannot actually make utilitarian calculations in an unbiased way. In health care this mode of reasoning could result in reductions in service, reduced standards of care, and the introduction of euthanasia, involuntary euthanasia, and infanticide if it could be argued that a greater number of individuals benefit than are harmed (Gillon 1992).

General utilitarianism

This is similar to act utilitarianism but incorporates the concept of Kant: when a decision is made one must consider what would happen if everyone did as they proposed (Beauchamp and Childress 1994).

Rule utilitarianism

This stresses that obedience to certain rules are fundamental to morality. Rules of conduct are established by calculating the greatest balance of good and evil. Emphasis is placed on keeping certain rules which produce the greatest good in the long term.

If, on balance, ignorance of distressing information protected a woman with breast cancer from gross psychological harm then, in spite of her personal desire to acquire knowledge, that knowledge could be withheld from her (Kerner 1990).

Merits of utilitarianism

- Utilitarianism claims to eliminate the mysterious and non-empirical. It is a secular philosophy and therefore not bound by religious precepts. Difficulties with the theory could therefore be suggested to be technical and not fundamental.
- If suffering is evil and happiness is good (Bentham 1948) then the aims of utilitarianism are clear: they are based on a linear continuum. It is suggested there are no competing principles as there are at times with deontology.
- Utilitarianism 'claims to provide a consistent and reliable procedure for making decisions in one or other variant of the hedonic calculus' (Gillon 1992).

Problems with utilitarianism

- It is possible for the situation to arise where an individual's needs are not met because the interests of the majority take priority (Glover 1990; Gillon 1992). An individual patient may request information but that request could be rejected because it is in the interests of others (e.g. clinicians, family, society, or science) not to disclose to the individual the full facts of her case. This can easily result in the 'individual versus society' conflict (Rawlings 1992).

  Another manifestation of this type of reasoning is the 'quality-adjusted life year'. This is a calculation to decide which treatments provide the greatest benefit to patients at the lowest cost. This means an operation like a hip replacement may have a high priority because it is relatively inexpensive, provides excellent surgical results, and enables an individual to enjoy many years of pain-free mobility, but a treatment like renal dialysis, which is expensive and non-curative, may not. Another facet to this is that only those who are known to benefit are offered treatment. This may mean that the elderly and patients with metastatic breast disease may not be selected for expensive treatment with a variable success rate.

- Utilitarianism may increase favourable consequences but those acting may be motivated by evil or immoral intentions. Utilitarianism can be seen as morally objectionable (Kerner 1990; Gillon 1992). It is possible for the innocent to suffer or for torture to be justified. Utilitarianism leaves out key elements like justice.

- Another difficulty is that utilitarian calculations cannot always be performed. Utilities are not always quantifiable. How can one judge which of two women with breast cancer is more valuable, needy, worthy, etc. and therefore should take precedence over the other. The consequences of a utilitarian action are not always simple to measure and evaluate (Gillon 1992).

It could be suggested that the application of one theory in every situation is not appropriate or adequate (Glover 1990; Calabresi and Bobbit 1978; Gillon 1992). Rules and principles often come into conflict. The analysis of principles is necessary in the context of a situation to see what is most applicable. It is important to consider alternatives and thereby weigh up their advantages and disadvantages. Decisions must be justified on the basis of appropriate principles or benefits of the expected outcome. The consequences must be fully considered, including legal consequences, for example some may feel a person with poor quality of life is better off dead but the law in the United Kingdom does not allow for voluntary or involuntary euthanasia.

Autonomy

Autonomy comes from the Greek 'autos' and 'nomos' meaning literally self-rule or self-government (Harris 1985). This has been interpreted as the ability to think, decide, or act freely without coercion or hindrance (Kirby 1983; Faulder 1985). Autonomy as a concept incorporates the notion of personhood (Aristotle 340 BC; Glover 1990; Benson 1983). Autonomy is an important concept when shared decision-making is considered. It accords to the individual the right to information which will enable him to make decisions about his own future.

Types of autonomy

There are many different types of autonomy and expressions of an individual's autonomy, e.g.:

- autonomy of thought: to make moral assessments or decisions
- autonomy of will: freedom to exercise one's will after due deliberation
- autonomy of action: ability to execute autonomy of thought and will.

Autonomy is rarely absolute. Individuals are restricted by law, social conditions, respect for the autonomy of others, finance health, etc. (Glover 1990).

Autonomy is determined by the individual's physical facilities. Environment plays a part in encouraging or discouraging autonomous behaviour. An individual must have the knowledge to pursue an end and select routes to that end, and they must be rational enough to select appropriate ends. With this in mind, how reasonable is it to expect any woman recently diagnosed with breast cancer to inform herself accurately about her disease, prognosis, proposed treatment options and their success/failure rates, then to weigh them up and finally after making a calculation of risk/benefit to come to a treatment decision (Thornton 1992)?

The principle of respect for autonomy

If a deontological perspective is adopted there is a moral requirement on us to respect the autonomy of others. This is generally accepted in Western society but limitations are imposed when there is potential harm to others and in a limited sense to oneself (Gillon 1992; Williams 1992). Kant argued that autonomy and respect for the autonomy of all other autonomous agents were features of rationality (1964, 1973). Mill suggested that respect for autonomy was necessary to maximize human welfare as long as no harm was caused to others and where the individuals respected possessed a degree of maturity (1962a,b).

How much autonomy does a person have to possess in order to be respected as a moral agent? Who decides how much autonomy a person possesses? In the case of the patient–clinician relationship it is the clinician who continues to make the decisions. Patients now have the right to access information (Department of Health 1992; NHS Executive Clinical Outcome Guidelines for Breast Cancer 1996) but this right has the proviso that if the clinician feels it is not in the patient's best interest physically or psychologically, this information can be withheld. Who is to make the judgements or decisions for those who are deemed to be non-autonomous or incompetent? Should we respect the autonomy of individuals in every case? Should respect for autonomy be maintained if it leads to harm for the individual? Should we respect the autonomy of the individual if it leads to harm for others? The British Medical Association sanctions the divulging of information concerning the diagnosis of acquired immune deficiency syndrome to the partners of those who are HIV positive on the grounds that harm may result if the partners cannot protect themselves. All these questions raise awareness that respect for autonomy is not always straightforward.

Harris (1985) discussed the issues surrounding the disclosure of false or incomplete information. If a patient is deliberately given false or incomplete information this could be seen as negating their personal autonomy. The fact that the issues surrounding autonomy are complex does not alter the fact that a mature, rational woman who has been diagnosed with breast cancer should have the facts of her case explained to her in the amount of detail she requests and should, in collaboration with her clinician, share in any decisions regarding her future treatment if she so wishes. This would be a tangible expression of respect for her autonomy (Maslin 1993; 1994; Fallowfield *et al.* 1987; 1990*a*, 1994 *a,b*).

Baum *et al.* (1988) summed up the view of many clinicians:

'Autonomy, however, is not the only ethical imperative that should be considered, and perhaps an exaggerated regard for this single principle will put at risk not only the practice of scientific medicine but the whole concept of the doctor–patient relationship. Traditionally, the duty of doctors is to do their best for their individual patients (now the consumer), to select according to their needs and desires. If doctors are to continue to have the duty of care they must also bear in mind the other ethical principles when they treat each patient. For example, non-maleficence: could informed consent come in to this category since further information and uncertainties are forced upon patients at a time when they are feeling most vulnerable? Justice: should information be given about treatments which, if available, would drain the resources of the health service so that future patients may have to remain untreated?'

The current trend in the United Kingdom and United States of America is to facilitate autonomy within the health care system (Department of Health 1992; Williams 1992). The primary aim of health care continues to be the creation of circumstances in which personal autonomy and the ability to thrive and persevere can be achieved in spite of the trauma suffered. The King's Fund (1996) stated:

'Individualized or patient-centred care involves as a fundamental principle, respect for a client's autonomy. The health professional works to empower the client through communication, information-giving, involvement in (or devolvement of) decision-making and support.'

The World Health Organization's (1977) definition of health states:

'Health is a state of complete physical, mental, and social well-being and not merely the absence of disease or infirmity.'

For many individuals, respect of their legitimate personal autonomy, however it is expressed, leads to enhanced mental well-being (Ingelfinger 1980; Kirby 1983; Thornton 1992).

The right to refuse

It is acknowledged that stages of collaboration exist when patients are involved in decision-making (Cancer Research Campaign 1983; Brooking 1989; Baum 1994; British Association of Surgical Oncology 1994). This can be expressed by rational adults choosing to exercise their autonomy by being proactive and taking their own decisions (Thornton 1992) or by deciding they want to pass the responsibility for decision-making on to a professional (Ingelfinger 1980).

A mentally competent adult has the right to refuse treatment and can take their own discharge contrary to medical advice. This refers to any kind of treatment, e.g. blood transfusions, surgery, or chemotherapy, except in the case of harm to others. A mentally competent adult can delegate their autonomy (Ingelfinger 1980; Cancer Research Campaign 1983). Most competent adults usually make treatment decisions in consultation with health care professionals. In the case of children, informed consent is requested from the parents or guardians. Children should also be consulted. Parents/guardians refusing treatment on behalf of a child may have their child made a ward of court if the treating clinicians feel treatment is in the best interest of the child. Likewise, emergency treatment can be carried out on unconscious patients if that is deemed to be in the patient's best interests. Relatives have no right in law to refuse life-saving treatment.

The majority of women diagnosed with early breast cancer are rational, mature adults who are able to express a view on their desire whether or not to be involved in decision-making about their disease (Maslin *et al.* 1993; Cancer Research Campaign 1996).

Informed consent

There is now significant public and professional interest on the issues of patient decision-making, access to information, and participation in the informed consent process (Wells 1986; Fallowfield *et al.* 1990*a,b*; Department of Health 1992; Klimowski 1992; Williams 1992; Maslin 1993;1994; Saunders *et al.* 1994).

'The public is demanding the right to make informed decisions in most areas of health care, but lay person and professional alike are finding difficulty in giving the phrase "informed consent" tangible practical meaning.' (Maslin 1994)

Saunders *et al.* (1994) summarize:

'The first mention for the need for informed consent in medical practice came from William Beaumont in 1833, and was enshrined in the personal code of ethics of the "father of experimental medicine", Claude Bernard, in 1856. But the public took little interest in the issue of consent, either in routine clinical practice or research, until after World War II when the horrendous experiments performed by Nazi doctors on the inmates of concentration camps came to light. The public outrage and disgust engendered by these atrocities led to the formulation of the Nuremberg Code in 1947, laying out guidelines for experimentation on humans. This was followed in 1964 by the Helsinki Declaration, last revised in 1989, which remains a code of ethics for those engaged in medical research on humans. Later statements include those by the Medical Research Council (1962, 1963), the British Medical Association (1981), and the Belmont Report of the National Commission for the Protection of Human Subjects of Biomedical and Behavioural Research (1978).'

It has been suggested informed consent is the right of every human being to determine what shall be done to his/her own body. Cardozo (1914) summed up:

'Every human being of adult years and sound mind has a right to determine what shall be done with his own body; a surgeon who performs an operation without the patient's consent commits assault.'

This concept implies respect for the autonomy of the individual. Faulder (1985) suggests this can be defined as the individual's freedom to decide his or her own goals. Inherent in this principle is the notion of personal responsibility'.

The term 'informed consent' is frequently used to denote the interaction which takes place when an individual consents to treatment or participation in research. Informed consent has several components. These include:

- that the person is mentally competent/mature enough to give consent
- that the consent is given freely without coercion
- that the person is given adequate information on which to base their decision (Kirby 1983; Royal College of Physicians of London 1986; 1990*a*,*b*).

During a medico-legal case (Salgo vs. Leland Stanford Junior Board of Trustees, 317 P 2d 170 [Cal 1957]) it was stated the doctor had a duty to inform a patient of 'any facts which are necessary to form the basis of an intelligent consent by the patient to the proposed treatment'. Unless a woman has access to relevant and accurate information about her disease, treatment, and prognosis, how can she exercise her autonomy and give consent to treatment in any meaningful way?

A number of ethical principles are employed when due accord is given to the practice of informed consent. These include respect for the person, truth telling, justice, and beneficence. The concept of 'informed consent' is an attempt to equalize or develop partnership in the relationship between clinician and patient by respecting the individual's autonomy (Kirby 1983).

Kennedy (1988) suggests it is the question of information which 'provokes the greatest discussion and raises the most difficult problem'. A clinician owes a duty of care to his patient. This duty includes informing the patient of the most appropriate course of treatment for that patient and all the information that he feels is necessary for a patient to make a decision. The clinician can argue that if provision of distressing information may be harmful to a patient, he may on his professional discretion omit to inform a patient fully. The clinician must however answer truthfully any question posed by the patient unless he deems it not to be in 'the patient's best interest' (Wells 1986).

'Should a doctor be found to have breached his duty to inform his patient, the patient may recover damages if he can prove that had he been given the information he would not have consented to treatment, and that he has suffered harm as a consequence in that a risk he was not warned of materialized.' (Kennedy 1988)

In the United States, women with breast cancer constitute a group of health consumers who have initiated more open communication. In several American states physicians are legally bound to inform patients with breast cancer about breast cancer (Gantz 1992).

'In these states, higher rates of breast-conserving surgery have been found, suggesting that patient participation in medical decision-making does have an effect on the type of treatment selected.' (Hack *et al.* 1994)

Kirby (1983) suggests an informed consent 'is that consent which is obtained after the patient has been adequately instructed about the ratio of risk and benefit involved in the procedure as compared to alternative procedures or no treatment at all'. Some would suggest (de Vahl Davis 1992) this is virtually impossible and pose the question 'Can professionals ever give enough information for patients really to know how they will feel if they consent to a procedure?'

Michael Baum has participated in the debate on informed consent for many years (Baum and Houghton 1988; Baum *et al.* 1988; Saunders and Baum 1993; Baum 1994). Baum (1995), after discussing the value of informed consent, argued:

'There are, however, arguments on the other side. How can consent be fully informed? How can the patient without the benefit of six years of training understand the disease, and for that matter understand the logic of scientific empiricism? If you tell a patient we are really uncertain whether treatment A is better than treatment B, you undermine his or her confidence. Doctors like to practise benificently. We do not like to frighten and alarm our patients. Yet when we do tell them our uncertainties and fully disclose to the patient the hazards of the disease itself and the hazards of the operation down to the finest detail, we cause them illness. We make them distressed and anxious.'

Some patients (Thornton 1992) argue strongly that patients often slip into stereotypical submissive roles when they interact with their clinicians and this is reinforced by the fact that they are in an unequal situation as far as possessing relevant information to make informed choices and decisions. Kirby (1983) states 'it is hard to define the expression "informed consent" in a way that will accommodate all the ramifications of interpersonal relationships that can arise in a dependent environment of health care'. It is for this reason other forms of information may be made available to equalize the patient information gap, e.g. literature, visual material, and audio recordings. Bond and Thomas (1992) suggests:

'In medicine, an increasing emphasis is being placed on consumer opinion with regard to what constitutes appropriate treatment. Doctors have realized that what constitutes desirable patient outcomes should not be left to professionals alone, but should be viewed in the light of patients' needs and wishes.'

It is the clinician who has the obligation to obtain informed consent but it is not a legal duty in the United Kingdom (World Medical Association Declaration of Helsinki 1964 [amendments 1975, 1983, 1989]; Kirby 1983; Baum 1986; Wells 1986; Department of Health 1992). This situation is further confused by the fact that nurses in the United Kingdom, particularly specialist nurses caring for patients with breast cancer, have taken on a role as information giver, advocate, and assistant in the treatment decision-making process (Royal College of Nursing 1977; Lazweski 1981; Cancer Research Campaign 1983; Copp 1986; Wells 1986; Fallowfield *et al.* 1990*a,b*; Maslin 1993, 1994). Melia (1985) stated that:

'Consent to medical treatment is not an area in which nurses can ever truly be held responsible. It would perhaps be not only prudent but also morally sound to recognize this fact and leave doctors' business to doctors. The handmaiden image, from which nurses are striving to free themselves, is in danger of coming back in to play in a positively dangerous way in the guise of a new-found professionalism and the call of teamwork.'

Melia's comments are hard to reconcile with this current onus on nurses, especially specialist nurses, to provide additional medical information to enable patients to make treatment decisions (Watson *et al.* 1988). This role and function is not straightforward and should never be taken on without appropriate education and support (Roberts and Fallowfield 1990). Melia correctly points out that if such functions are taken on by nurses they must be prepared to be legally responsible for their actions (1986).

Wells (1986) suggested 'Too often we make assumptions about the ability of patients to understand what is being told to them and this leads doctors and nurses unwittingly (or otherwise) to keep important information from them'. In the United States the concept of the 'prudent patient' (Canterbury vs. Spence, The 'Prudent Patient' Standard, 464 F 2d [DC1972]) has been adopted, attempting to incorporate in law the view of the intelligent average patient when trying to assess if a patient has been adequately informed. Kirby (1983) strongly supported, however, the notion that if a patient did not wish to be informed this must be respected as this in itself is the expression of the patient's autonomy. Autonomy can be exercised by the individual but it can also be delegated by the individual to her clinician.

Clinicians and nurses are expected to ensure patients are able to make informed choices when they consider conventional surgery or treatment options (Faulder 1985; Melia 1985; Copp 1986). Patients are also demanding the right to give or refuse consent to participation in clinical trials which may or may not benefit them, directly based on full disclosure of information (Cancer Research Campaign 1983; Copp 1986; Baum and

Houghton 1988; Tobias 1988; Feinmann 1988; Faulder 1992; Maslin 1993; 1994), but how can this requirement be met equitably and to the satisfaction of all concerned? Baum (1982, 1994) argued strongly that the management of carcinoma of the breast has been one of the most hotly debated subjects among surgeons in modern times. Patients are often not aware of the many areas of uncertainty and debate in the treatment of their disease. This raises the issue of how, without readily available information in an acceptable format for the lay person, can a patient be able to participate in decision-making.

Maslin *et al.* (1993) aimed to survey, by self-completed questionnaires, the experiences and opinions of 300 randomly selected women (100 cancer patients in a clinical trial, 100 non-cancer patients in a clinical trial, and 100 patients not involved in a clinical trial) attending a breast unit, of their experiences when being asked to give consent to join a clinical trial and their opinions as to what they would consider appropriate to be able to give 'informed consent'.

The results indicated a number of areas in which the women were satisfied with the provision of information and support, e.g. having good verbal/written information and having time to reflect prior to making any decision, and also areas where improvements could be made, e.g. having more explicit information on side-effects of drugs and treatment. When the patients expressed their views on their requirements in relation to information and support, over 90% of the women responding wanted access to all the information and support listed, including verbal and written information, an indication of personal time commitment to the clinical trial, an outline of information the trial would produce, information on possible and probable side-effects, physical and emotional discomforts, and withdrawal rights, and also ongoing information and support throughout treatment (Maslin 1994).

Kirby (1983) suggested 'A recurrent feature of our civilization is said to be respect for the autonomy of the individual human being "with inherent dignity and value"'. This respect for the autonomy of the individual is now being given tangible expression by allowing patients access to all the material facts which have a bearing on their medical and nursing care (Department of Health 1992; Gillon 1992; Silverman and Altman 1996). The mechanism of informed consent (Kirby 1983; Royal College of Physicians 1990*a,b*) is also a safeguard to this autonomy.

Informed consent has been summed up as 'adequate disclosure from the informant met by adequate understanding from the person receiving the information, thus enabling the latter freely to give or refuse her consent' (Faulder 1985). This description begs the question of what is adequate and who decides when this has been achieved? Where is the balance of power to be held—by the clinician or the patient? If patients demand the right to make these decisions, are they always prepared to accept the corresponding responsibilities of their decisions? The situation could arise where a patient's considered decision results in harm to them which may have been prevented if the clinician's advice had been taken.

Schafer (1989) argues strongly:

'Every potential research subject is legally and morally entitled to assess the risks and benefits of participating in a clinical trial. The procedure of informed consent is the mechanism whereby the patient becomes a partner in the enterprise rather than a mere guinea pig.'

Many patients with breast cancer are given the opportunity to take part in clinical trials (Williams 1992; Maslin 1993; Saunders *et al.* 1994; Baum 1994; 1995). If researchers wish to address the issues of breast cancer prevention and cure, they need the cooperation and commitment of the women from whom they recruit information, and collaboration appear to be fundamental to this relationship for many women (Fallowfield *et al.* 1990*a,b*; Maslin 1993).

Acts and omissions

The concept of acts and omissions with reference to informed consent may be relevant. Clough (1977) suggested that there is a difference between an act with the intention to harm and an omission which may result in harm but where the intention was to do good 'Thou shalt not kill but needst not strive officiously to keep alive.' It can be argued that an individual, e.g. a clinician, may not be able to foresee all the results of his actions, therefore he cannot be blamed unless he acted without due care and attention. A clinician may feel that by omitting to tell a patient unpleasant information he is acting in her best interest by attempting to preserve her psychological state. This may result in the patient's trust being broken when the full situation is known. On the other hand, a clinician may act in what he feels is his patient's best interest, giving her full information to consent to treatment, only to find that the result is severe psychiatric morbidity for the patient (Tobias 1988).

Advocacy

Advocacy encapsulates the concept of sharing information, allowing the patient to decide on their own course of action and then enabling the patient to realize that decision by offering the patient whatever support or resources they need to achieve their aim (Wells 1986). Often nurses take up the role of patient advocate (Wells 1986; Bird 1994) when patients face making decisions or exercising choices. Some have questioned the notion of nurses being used as patient advocates. Historically, nurses have been subservient to their medical colleagues. The bureaucratic structure they were a part of did not encourage questioning, deviation, or advocacy. They were often seen as the handmaidens who carried out medical prescriptions and instructions.

Wells (1986) suggested:

'Rarely, if ever, is the role of the nurse considered. Perhaps this is because of a belief held by many of our medical colleagues that a nurse who is fully involved may be unable to remain impartial and unemotive in the care of sick people. One voice in the veritable wilderness was that of the Cancer Research Campaign Working Party in Breast Conservation: "Ideally, the trained nurse counsellor, or some other suitably qualified person, should help obtain informed consent".'

Since Maguire *et al.* (1978, 1980) established that nurses appropriately trained in assessment for psychiatric morbidity could successfully identify patients at risk and make appropriate referrals to a department of psychological medicine, nurses, especially clinical nurse specialists in breast care, have been taking a leading role in acting as advocates for patients diagnosed with breast cancer (Maguire *et al.* 1980; Maguire and Faulkner 1988*b*). This role has been evaluated by the work of Watson *et al.* (1988)

and Roberts and Fallowfield (1990), and supported by advisory documents such as the Forrest Report (1986), Cancer Relief Macmillan Fund's Minimum Standards for Breast Care (1994), the British Association of Surgical Oncologists' guidelines on treatment protocols (1994), and the British Breast Group's assessment of specialist cancer centres (1994), all of which have endorsed the supportive role of appropriately trained specialist nurses who are able to participate in information-giving, decision-making, and psychological support.

The United Kingdom Central Council for Nursing, Midwifery, and Health Visitors (UKCC) state in their document *Exercising Accountability* 'the role of patient's advocate is an essential aspect of good professional nursing practice' (UKCC 1989), but it is interesting to note that the UKCC go on to say in the same document that other health care professionals, not only the nurse, can also be the patient's advocate. This could be problematic if every discipline feels they are the body acting on the patient's behalf. This also raises another issue. Is advocacy a function which is taken on in any given instance? For example, a woman has just been given a diagnosis of breast cancer and she is being pressed to make a treatment decision; a nurse who is present sees the woman's distress and in this instance acts as an advocate to assist the woman to remedy the situation. Or is it an ongoing relationship? For example, just before an individual patient receives a diagnosis of breast cancer she is introduced to her breast care nurse who will be available to her at any time, anywhere, and throughout her disease continuum.

It has been argued that several unwarranted assumptions are inherent in the role of nurse advocates: Are nurses capable of abrogating their vested interests as professionals and challenging the vested interests to colleagues? Will society allow the sick true autonomy? Nurses can be seen as professionals in an institutional setting involved as agents of social control assisting doctors. Do nurses have a vested interest in maintaining the exclusive professional power of the establishment on which they depend for employment? If nurses act as patient advocates, are they not fostering a relationship in which the patient can develop a dependency? Advocacy could be used as a vehicle for paternalism (Bird 1994) Advocacy may result in schism, and conflict with the nurse and patient being seen as colluding. It could be argued nurses are not trained to plead the cause of others and therefore independent advocates or counsellors should be made available to patients.

Advocates need to be articulate, self-aware, and professional. Advocates require specific knowledge, skills, and motivation to facilitate the patient in their quest. They must be able to function within the health care system but not be compromised by it (Copp 1986). The advocate must put the client's interests impartially above his own. He must be emotionally neutral towards his client as far as sex, creed, colour, and status are concerned.

Wells (1986) argued 'Nurses can only have the right to a role in the giving of informed consent if they have sufficient know-ledge and emotional equilibrium to express a rational informed opinion'. He went on to argue 'If nurses become involved in informed consent, as many people believe they should, and par-ticipate equally with their colleagues in the role, they must be seen to be less emotional, more knowledgeable, and mature in their discussions and opinions; and if they achieve that they may well lay aside the dictum of Mallett that "she [the nurse] must never ask why, and seldom, if ever, ask how"'.

Rationale for advocacy

Advocacy is a tangible expression of respect for the notion of patient autonomy. It also recognizes the fact that some patients may have diminished autonomy. The nature of relationships within the National Health Service is not equal. It could be sug-gested that the doctor–patient relationship lacks equality, hence the need for advocacy to put forward the patient's point of view. This is necessary in order to fulfil the duty owed to patients of justice and beneficence. Patients have legal and moral rights which must be protected.

3

Clinical effectiveness and evidence-based practice

Anna M. Maslin

Even if an argument is forcefully made for a woman with breast cancer having the right to information which will enable her to exercise her autonomy if she so wishes by being involved in the decision-making process, how likely will it be that accurate, clinically effective, individualized information will be available for her? This section aims to briefly review the position in relation to breast cancer.

People living in the 20th century are living with a degree of fear and a vast amount of uncertainty (Read 1995). This applies equally to issues current in society: politics, religion, ethics, and health care. Richards *et al.* (1993) stated:

'Marked cultural changes have occurred in Europe and the USA over the past 30 years, with an increasing concern for individual autonomy and the rights of the consumer. Changes in medical practice have occurred which reflect these broader changes in society. Increasing emphasis is now placed on the provision of information to patients and their participation in decision-making about their management.'

But how can women facing a diagnosis of breast cancer truly participate when there are so many factors, including a knowledge deficit on the patient's part, variations in clinical practice (sometimes evidence based, sometimes not), and variations in availability, added to the impact of stress and selective perception on a vulnerable patient (Roper *et al.* 1988; Coates and Simes 1992; Baum 1995; Beaver *et al.* 1996)?

Saunders *et al.* (1994) observed that:

'The practice of medicine has always been 'experimental': cures being tried on patients and the results observed. Traditionally, therapeutic regimens were derived from anecdotal experience, and medical innovations were largely a matter of trial and error. Such was the discovery of Ambroise Pare in 1537 of a new dressing for gunshot wounds. Prior to all this, all authorities had taught that burning oil should be applied to the wound to counteract the poison. But in his first campaign he was so inundated with gunshot wounds that he was forced to use an alternative "digestive" made of egg yolks, oil of roses, and turpentine: "That night I could not sleep at my ease ... I raised myself early to visit them, when beyond my hope I found those to whom I had applied the digestive medicament felling little pain, their wounds neither swollen nor inflamed, and having slept throughout the night. The others whom I had applied the boiling oil were feverish with much pain and swelling."'

Baum (1994) states:

'It is indeed a cosy myth that the doctor knows best for every patient, for every disease. A peculiar conspiracy of the public and profession together has effectively held back the progress of medicine for 100 years, delaying its entry into the scientific era and making it extraordinarily difficult to draw the line of demarcation between orthodox and "alternative" medicine.'

Michael Peckham at the time he was NHS Director of Research and Development supported this view. He stated 'Some interventions which were used with genuine conviction in the past have been shown over time to be ineffective or harmful' (Moran 1995).

Kee (1996) summarizes:

'Patients today demand more information about their treatment. Doctors, however, seem reluctant to cast aside ingrained habits of paternalism, believing they can best interpret therapeutic choices for their patients. Whether doctors can be more objective and effective than patients in interpreting the probabilities of medical evidence is open to question. On the other hand, the exercise of choice by patients may itself have a bearing on probabilities of outcome. Involving patients more in making therapeutic choices is justified if doctors can present options in an unbiased and effective manner and if the process improves the outcome of the care delivered.'

Baum (1982) and Schafer (1989) rightly draw attention to the fact that many patients are unaware how many clinicians choose treatments based on their training and personal anecdotal experience. Clinical decisions are not always made based on empirical research but sometimes on 'trial and error'. Schafer (1989) states 'Many patients are unaware of the extent to which uncertainty pervades modern medicine'. Many patients and lay writers will question the ethics of randomized controlled trials but do not question the ethics of recommending untested treatments. Revealing the uncertainty which actually exists can often be as difficult for the patient as for the clinician. This difficulty is compounded when the clinician, in an effort to discover optimal treatments, is involved in clinical trials. In this situation the patient may feel she wishes to challenge his motives. Is the clinician now acting with her best interests at heart or with a research motive in mind (Schafer 1989)?

Roper *et al.* (1988) stated:

'Although modern medicine provides great benefits to large numbers of people, medical professionals and clinical researchers have expressed concern about the effectiveness and appropriateness of many current and emerging medical practices. For example, the evidence substantiating the effectiveness of many such practices is questionable and in many instances entirely lacking ... Many physicians lack the skills to interpret and critically evaluate medical literature, and they approach the same clinical problem with different theoretical assumptions, contributing to wide variations in practice patterns.'

Rawlings (1992) summarizes a possible scenario when a competent adult visits a physician:

'An individual with a problem consults a physician. Skilful interviewing, examination, and selection of appropriate tests lead to rapid and accurate diagnosis of the problem.

The physician recommends a course of action: traditional historical experience, pharmacological study, and animal experiments have suggested certain approaches. Their comparative worth will have been verified clinically by appropriate human trials, and the physician will be aware of results through education, publication, and conferences, and thus be able to judge what to recommend to the patient and accurately describe the alternatives.

The patient decides: full, honest, and reliable information, given in the context of a relationship of trust and confidence, allows the patient to choose the most personally suitable treatment plan.

The plan is implemented: an educated, motivated, cooperative health care team work with the patient to carry out what has been decided. Funds and facilities are available to do this in the way intended.'

Rawlings (1992) goes on to say:

'It can readily be appreciated that we have a long way to go to achieve this ideal in the 1990s. What is more vexing, and gives rise to the profoundly difficult questions of human experimentation, is that the validity of most recommended approaches is in dispute. Personal anecdotal experience, published historical results, conjecture based on results in animal or possibly comparable diseases are the usual reasons for outlining a certain treatment plan (as well as . . . an unquestioning belief in what was taught in medical school or residency). These justifications for therapeutic decisions are grossly inadequate to assess the worth of manoeuvres which will have such an impact on human lives.'

Evidence-based medicine aimed to be a new paradigm for medical practice which 'de-emphasizes intuition, unsystematic clinical experience, and pathophysiologic rationale as sufficient grounds for clinical decision-making and stresses the examination of evidence from clinical research (EBM Working Group 1992). 'The term "evidence-based medicine" (EBM) or, more broadly, evidence-based clinical practice reflects the aspiration that doctors and other clinical professionals should pursue their work of diagnosis, therapy, and care on the basis of procedures which are known through research evidence to be effective' (Long and Harrison 1996). The phrase "evidence-based medicine" attempts to encapsulate the concept of a process of lifelong, problem-based learning in which caring for patients creates the need for evidence about diagnosis, prognosis, therapy, and other clinical and health care issues.

In the EBM process:

• these information needs are turned into answerable questions
• the best evidence from which to answer them (whether from clinical examination, the diagnostic laboratory, published literature, or other sources) are tracked down
• evidence is critically appraised for its validity and usefulness; the results of this appraisal are applied in clinical practice, and
• the outcome is evaluated.

EBM has caused a great deal of discussion within the medical profession. There are some for whom EBM has always been a priority (Baum 1982; 1990; 1995; Baum *et al.* 1988). As previously stated, Baum (1982) suggested 'It would shatter the image of a noble and caring profession if the public were aware of how much "medical treatment" could easily be looked upon as uncontrolled experimentation'. Baum (1995), however, notes that the responsible doctor 'bases his decision first and foremost on the quality of the evidence and that this intervention will be advantageous for the patient'. Baum (1995) stated:

'It is possible to construct a hierarchy of approaches to the development of knowledge in medicine. The weakest kind of evidence is anecdotal. This includes anecdotal case reports, and even a report of a series of cases without adequate controls. The strongest evidence comes from the randomized controlled trial, ideally the confirmed or replicated randomized controlled trial.'

Naylor (1995), when discussing those who are sceptical about EBM, stated:

'A backlash is not surprising in view of the inflated expectations of outcomes orientated and evidence-based medicine and the fears of some clinicians that these concepts threaten the art of patient care. Evidence-based medicine offers little help in many of the grey zones of practice where the evidence about risk–benefit ratios of competing clinical options is incomplete or contradictory.'

This is an important issue in breast cancer care (Coates and Simes 1992). Breast cancer is often a chronic, unpredictable disease and, in spite of consistent research endeavour, there remain areas in which there is more than one treatment of choice, and those treatments do not carry an absolute guarantee of success thus necessitating an evaluation by the clinician and/or patient of the risks and benefits (British Association of Surgical Oncology 1994; British Breast Group 1994; NHS Executive Clinical Outcomes Group 1996*a,b*).

Rawlings (1992) points out that what may be considered the 'best' treatment in terms of length of life may have unacceptable side-effects which would impinge on quality of life. Even if a 'best' treatment was known, it is sometimes the case that the results of research are not known by individual practitioners or accepted by them. Another key factor is that the patients' priorities and values when considering treatment may vary considerably to the clinicians' (Cassileth *et al.* 1980). This discussion becomes particularly pertinent when one considers the patient with cancer. For many adult cancers, including breast cancer, cure rates are poor. Surgery and treatments offered are often disfiguring and complex with debilitating side-effects. Those patients who wish to participate in their treatment decisions require clear, concise but full information to enable them to make a relevant choice (Fallowfield *et al.* 1994*b*). Women with breast cancer are often facing a future with a chronic disease in which there are few guarantees. This is compounded by the fact that there is legitimate debate regarding the management of breast cancer (Baum 1982; Fallowfield *et al.* 1989; Powles and Smith 1991; Rubens 1992; Saunders and Baum 1994; Rijken *et al.* 1995), adding difficulty to the decision-making process. Women with breast cancer are in a unique position: they face choices and decisions relating to local and systemic therapy which are often complex and uncertain, but they and their clinicians do have access to a very comprehensive portfolio of research-based evidence on which to base therapeutic decisions (Baum *et al.* 1988; Baum 1990; Powles and Smith 1991; Fisher *et al.* 1989*b*; 1993; Harris *et al.* 1993; Fisher and Anderson 1994). There is concern over how uncertainty is communicated to patients. Goldie (1982) astutely commented:

'Obviously one would not begin to seek out and display the truth without undertaking to remain with patients whilst they digested and assimilated it: to do otherwise would be like performing a skilful surgical operation and then leaving the skin unsecured.'

Women with small, uncomplicated, localized breast cancers do have a choice of surgical treatment options (Fisher *et al.* 1989*b*; Fallowfield *et al.* 1990*a,b*). Jacobson *et al.* (1996) reported 'Breast-conserving surgery plus radiation therapy was as effective as mastectomy'. This has obviously been known for some time (Fisher *et al.* 1989*b*) but it does draw attention to the fact that women in this group are able to exercise a genuine choice based on evidence. Evidence also shows us that women when offered a choice will not always opt for breast-conserving surgery and that psychiatric morbidity is experienced in both surgical groups (Fallowfield *et al.* 1986; 1990*a,b*).

4

Communication, psychiatric morbidity, access to information, and decision-making

A.M. Maslin

Considerable research has been carried out in relation to the psychiatric morbidity experienced by women diagnosed with breast cancer (Maguire 1988; 1990; Maguire *et al.* 1980; 1982; 1983; Watson *et al.* 1988). It is known that approximately one in four women with breast cancer will suffer from severe anxiety and or depression requiring psychiatric intervention (Maguire *et al.* 1980; Watson *et al.* 1988). It is also now known that the communication, or lack of it, between breast cancer patients and their clinicians has a psychological impact and affects the patients' ability to adjust (Fallowfield *et al.* 1986; 1987; 1990*a,b*; 1994*a,b*). This chapter reviews the impact of communication on psychiatric morbidity and the role choice plays in adjustment to breast cancer diagnosis and treatment.

Maguire and colleagues have looked extensively at the communication and assessment skills exhibited by clinicians and nurses (Maguire 1990; Maguire *et al.* 1978; 1980; 1984; 1986). It is important that clinicians and nurses dealing with patients affected by a cancer diagnosis are able to communicate the information the patient requires as effectively as possible (Maguire and Faulkner 1988*a*). It is also important that the people involved in information giving and psychological support are able to assess the impact of the information on the patient, and psychiatric morbidity (Maguire *et al.* 1980; Maguire and Faulkner 1988*b*; Maguire 1990).

Maguire and colleagues (Maguire *et al.* 1980; 1982; 1983; 1984) developed an assessment tool and communication workshops from their extensive research into teaching communication skills (Maguire 1985; 1990). They also looked at the communication skills of clinicians (Maguire 1985) and nurses (Maguire *et al.* 1980) and found that without appropriate training their skills were often deficient. Doctors, in the past, were often unaware of the deficiency. Although there is now a greater awareness of the psychological and information needs of cancer patients, it would appear that the training and supervision of 'cancer counsellors' varies considerably (Roberts and Fallowfield 1990). Roberts (1990, p. 33), commenting on a nursing sample surveyed, noted that:

'Only a third . . . (33.9%) used a particular counselling scheme or model in their work. This might reflect the low percentage of respondents with recognized formal counselling/psychotherapy qualifications . . . Formal assessment of clients was carried out by only 23.4% of respondents.'

Watson *et al.* (1984, p. 2008) noted that denial is used as a coping mechanism by some women diagnosed with breast cancer, and that those 'who denied the seriousness of a cancer diagnosis, experienced significantly less mood disturbance'. Maguire agrees that some patients will use sublimation or denial as a coping mechanism and that that mode of action may be appropriate, but he also acknowledges that there are some patients who want 'more or complete information' (Maguire 1990). Maguire and Faulkner (1988c, p. 974) suggest:

'Patients use denial when the truth is too painful to bear. So denial should not be challenged unless it is creating serious problems for the patient or relative. In challenging denial it is important to do so gently so that fragile defences are not disrupted but firmly enough so that any awareness can be explored or developed'.

The skill lies in the professional's ability to discern the information requirements of the patient and to explain the way forward, including advantages and disadvantages, in such a way that the patient is able to participate to the level they wish (Maguire *et al.* 1978; Maguire and Faulkner 1988c).

In an unusually small (*n*=40) study by Shapiro *et al.* (1992) using video-taped consultations, it was observed that the expression and demeanour of the oncologist, i.e. whether he looked worried or not when giving information to the patient, affected the patient's response and ability to recall clinical information.

Patients who saw a worried oncologist perceived the clinical situation to be worse, reported significantly higher levels of anxiety, and had significantly higher pulse rates.

Fallowfield *et al.* (1986), in a study which randomized patients with no strong treatment preference to mastectomy or breast conservation, noted anxiety in 33% of those who underwent mastectomy and found 38% of those who underwent breast conservation had an anxiety state, depressive illness, or both. This study, though useful, did not fully take into account the possible bias that is introduced by including data from women who were willing to be randomized to either breast conservation or mastectomy. Fallowfield *et al.* (1990*b*, p. 1394), in a follow-up study which addressed these issues, discussed the impact of patients being allowed choice. They concluded that

'Whatever the treatment for early breast cancer, good communication skills at the initial 'bad news' consultation, when diagnosis and management are discussed, may well contribute much to future adjustment'.

Dr Maureen Roberts was Clinical Director of the Edinburgh Breast Screening project from 1979 to 1989. Dr Roberts was diagnosed with breast cancer and subsequently died of the disease. She said:

'Communication is all important. Proper truthful accounts of diagnosis, treatment and aftercare must be written and made available everywhere, so that women become well informed and most important, start to take part in the decision making process for themselves (Roberts 1998)'.

If it is accepted that (a) sentient adult women with breast cancer have a right to express their autonomy, if they so wish, by accessing well-communicated and accurate evidence-based information relating to their disease and treatment options and that (b) this may be positive for their future psychological adjustment, how likely is that to be their experience?

Goldie (1982) commented 'The question whether or not to tell the patient the truth usually arises in connection with cancer'. He suggested that healthcare professionals were often influenced by their own fantasies of what it must be like to have cancer, and that they often adopted a policy of avoiding mentioning unpleasant or distressing news for as long as possible. This alleged behaviour on the part of healthcare professionals may still, in part, be correct, but it needs to be counterbalanced with the fact that many patients, in particular breast cancer patients, have adopted a more proactive stance in relation to their own health care and related issues (Kfir and Slevin 1991; Richards *et al.*1995; Cancer Relief Macmillan Fund 1994; Hack *et al.* 1994; Maslin 1994; Kee 1996).

Kfir and Slevin (1991, p. 19) argued that information means control and power. They suggested 'Information is a major asset when trying to create a new order and less chaos'. This ability to feel in control is a coping mechanism for some patients. Hack *et al.* (1994, p. 280) suggest:

'Two important ways by which cancer patients gain a sense of control over their illness include (a) acquiring information about their illness and its treatment and (b) playing a more active role in decision-making. Patients' feelings of psychological control over their health may also increase if they perceive that their needs for medical information have been satisfied. Conversely, psychological control may be defined as the belief that one can predict what will occur in the environment and that one can modify the environment to produce change which is fundamental to successful adaptation'.

This promotion of active participation in decision-making must, however, be balanced by the fact that a patient seeking advice about a suspected cancer is under considerable stress (Hughes 1993; Luker *et al.* 1995). The individual is suddenly faced with a number of very real difficulties: first they must see their family doctor and be referred to a specialist in their field, then begin to learn a new language relating to their disease and possible treatments, next come to terms with their diagnosis, decide whether they are comfortable with the advice of their specialist, and decide whether to seek a second opinion. Finally, some patients have to make a choice between various treatment options. All these decisions can put patients under considerable stress. The decisions they make at this time may literally have an impact on whether they live or die (Valanis and Rumpler 1985). Maslin (1993) noted that when patients were questioned about which aspects of the information were inadequate, they often mentioned that at the time of the breast cancer diagnosis they were in a state of shock and could not therefore take in or comprehend much of what the clinician said.

Health care professionals express a variety of views on whether or not patients should be actively involved in decisions relating to their care (Cassileth *et al.* 1980; Wagener and Taylor 1986; Tobias 1988; Fallowfield *et al.* 1990*a,b*, 1994*a,b*; Waterworth and Luker 1990; Baum 1994; Beaver *et al.* 1996; Curtis and Lacey 1996; Mort 1996). Baum (1995) stated

'Decision making in medical practice is a complicated algorithm. A therapeutic decision is made as a result of a dialogue between the doctor and the patient. The doctor and the patient approach this decision making through different pathways. The patient has expectations and priorities, some of which may be unrealistic. For instance, he or she may prefer to trade quality of life for length of life or vica versa. The patient has fears. These may be rational or irrational, and patients of mine in the past have been so frightened of surgery that they have refused that advice. Finally, patients, to varying degrees, wish to express autonomy, and autonomy is expressed through involvement in the decision making process. Clinicians on the other hand are weighing up their own scales of merit. There is the quality of the evidence known to them, the availability of the best treatment locally or nationally, there is the influence of their own ethics and subliminal preferences'.

Rawlings (1992, p. 29) stated 'the way we conceptualise medical care has been changing; we no longer see the patient only as a passive recipient of medical intervention, but also as a client/partner in a mutual enterprise of seemingly ever-expanding scope.' It is this premise that underpins much of the thinking surrounding patient access to information (Maslin 1993, 1994; Saunders *et al.* 1994). There are the ethical/moral reasons why patients should be able to access the information they require, but there is also a change in public opinion. Breast cancer patients in particular are demanding their rights as thinking individuals and consumers of healthcare (Richards *et al.* 1995). The Patients' Charter (1992) has made explicit for many patients the fact that they have recognized rights within the National Health Service. Goldie (1982, p. 128) suggested that the moral issue is not simply whether or not to tell cancer patients the truth, but more importantly how to do so. 'Time and trouble is needed to understand patients and help them understand their situation'.

Clinicians, scientists, and nurses are in a difficult position. They must strike a sensitive balance between providing adequate explanation and not causing the patient undue worry by providing unsolicited and perhaps frightening information. (World Medical Association Declaration of Helsinki 1964; Cancer Research Campaign Working Party on Breast Conservation 1983; Baum 1986). This puts them into the position of having to balance patient rights with healthcare professionals' duties (Schafer 1989; Rawlings 1992; Maslin 1993, 1994). Wagener and Taylor (1986) noted that in failed transplant patients, health professionals recalled the circumstances of the initial decision in a manner that lessened personal responsibility for it. In that way they were able to rationalize to themselves that they had no choice but to take that course of action and therefore they were not personally responsible for it.

Patients with cancer have been found to express different opinions on the quantity/quality of information they would find desirable and on whether they wish to be actively involved in treatment decisions (Ingelfinger 1980; Baum and Houghton 1988; Tobias 1988; Beisecker and Beisecker 1990; Thornton 1992; Maslin 1993, 1994). It is common in the clinical oncology situation for a patient to say initially that they want to be told all the relevant information regarding their case and then for them to be unable or unwilling to hear (Priestman 1986; Maslin 1993).

Cassileth *et al.* (1980), in a survey of 256 patients with cancer, found that at about 10 months post diagnosis 95% of patients wanted to know whether or not they had cancer, 'what the treatment would accomplish', and 'what the likelihood of cure is'. Approximately 80% wanted 'as much information as possible' and about 60% felt having that information was absolutely essential.

Strull *et al.* (1984) found, when surveying 210 hypertensive outpatients, that 41% of patients wanted more information about hypertension. In 29% of cases the clinician overestimated the amount of information the patient wanted. They also note the fact that clinicians thought 78% of their patients wished to participate in decision-making when in fact only 53% wished to. They found the fact that a patient chose not to take the initial therapeutic decision did not mean they did not wish to participate in the ongoing evaluation of therapy.

Sutherland *et al.* (1989, p. 260) conducted a similar but smaller study ($n = 52$) with cancer patients, but in their study 77% of the patients said they had participated in decision-making to the level they wished. Most of the remaining 23% would have liked a greater opportunity to participate. Although the patients sought information, a majority, 63%, preferred the clinician to make the therapeutic decision for them.

Fallowfield *et al.* (1986) reported that more than half the women with breast cancer in a UK randomized study felt they had been given inadequate information when the various therapeutic options were discussed.

Blanchard *et al.* (1988) found out of 439 encounters between hospitalized adult cancer patients and their doctors, 92% of patients preferred to receive all information, whether good or bad, and 69% indicated they wanted full participation in their care.

Beisecker and Beisecker (1990, p. 19) noted in their study with 106 rehabilitation patients, looking at information-seeking behaviours, that patients desired information about a wide rage of medical topics, but did not engage in many information-seeking behaviours when communicating with doctors. While the patients desired information, they regarded the doctors as 'the appropriate persons to make medical decisions.' Patients whose conversations with the doctor lasted longer than 19 minutes began to display more information seeking behaviour.

Suominen (1992) found that out of 109 breast cancer patients, 54% said they should have a significant share in decisions about their treatment and most, 64%, were dissatisfied with the information they received.

Luker *et al.* (1993), looking at 150 newly diagnosed women with breast cancer, found 20% wished to actively participate in the decision-making about their breast cancer treatment, 28% wished to be involved and share in the decision regarding their future treatment, and 52% wished to leave the decision-making to their clinicians.

Hack, Degner and Dyck (1994) studied breast cancer patients' preferences for involvement in treatment decisions and preferences for information about diagnosis, treatment, side-effects, and prognosis. They found women who desired an active role in treatment decision-making also desired detailed information. This relationship was less clear in passive patients (p. 135). Maslin (1993, 1994), Luker *et al.* (1995), and Richards *et al.* (1995) all point out that a desire for information may or may not result in the patient wanting to participate in treatment decision-making. Patients may exercise their autonomy by putting their confidence and trust in a clinician to make decisions on their behalf (Ingelfinger 1980; Degner and Sloane 1992).

Luker *et al.* (1995) supported nurses, particularly clinical nurse specialists, playing a key role in providing breast cancer patients with useful and appropriate information. In their study of 150 women newly diagnosed with breast cancer and 200 with benign breast disease, they found the top three information needs of the women with breast cancer were likelihood of cure, spread of disease, and treatment options. Luker *et al.* (1995) suggested this level of information was not within the scope of the average ward nurse but may well fall within the scope and practice of the specialist breast care nurse.

Bilodeau and Degner (1996) conducted a study with 74 women recently diagnosed with breast cancer to attempt to describe their preferred and actual roles in treatment decision-making. Of the group, 57% assumed a passive role in decision-making, although 43% stated this was their preference. Although 37% preferred a collaborative role, only 19% were able to achieve this. Bilodeau and Degner felt women who wish to collaborate in decision-making may find difficulty in achieving this aim. They strongly suggested that nurses can 'assess women's desired roles in treatment decision making and facilitate women achieving their preferred roles'.

Breast cancer survey—BACUP, Autumn 1995

Cancer BACUP (the British Association of Cancer United Patients) conducted a small survey to find out about the experience of breast cancer patients—users of BACUP Information Service. The questions were addressed to people with breast cancer, 18% of those who contact BACUP Information Service, for two weeks in Autumn 1995.

It should be emphasized that the sample was very small and unrepresentative. The majority of BACUP users are referred by health professionals and/or are strongly motivated to search for information. Consequently, they cannot represent in any way the whole population of people with breast cancer. Therefore, the survey only gives an indication of the way some users of BACUP were treated.

A) Who first told them and where was it?

The vast majority of breast cancer patients, 80%, were told by a consultant surgeon (specialist registrar), while only 5% were told by their GP.

Person that gave the diagnosis	(%)
Consultant/surgeon (including registrar)	80
GP	5
Other (including unspecified doctors)	15

75% were in an 'appropriate' place, such as a room with privacy or a consultant's or doctor's office when they were given their diagnosis. However, 13% were told in a ward or at home over the phone.

Place when given diagnosis	(%)
Room with privacy	41
Consultant's/doctor's office	34
Ward/at home over the phone	13
Other (not specified)	12

B) How long did they spend together?

Many patients, 37%, spent between 15 and 29 minutes with the health professional, whereas 27% spent between 5 and 14 minutes.

Time (minutes)	(%)
<5 minutes	14
5–14 minutes	27
15–29 minutes	37
⩾30	13
Other	9

C) What information they received when they were first told?

Almost half, 47%, of breast cancer patients received what they believed to be satisfactory information when they were given their original diagnosis. 58% received at least some information. A very high percentage, 42%, did not receive any information at all.

Information given	(%)
No information at all	42
Some information (not specified)	11
Yes, they had information	47

Of those that were given information and specified what it was precisely (47%), 70% had information about their cancer, treatment, and surgery issues. A lower proportion, 20%, were given BACUP booklets or information, and only 13% received information for counselling services.

Specific information	(%)
Cancer (including site specific, treatment and surgery information)	70
Counselling services	13
Booklets/leaflets (not specified)	10
BACUP booklets/information	10

D) What information would have found useful to receive when they were first told?

Not surprisingly, many people with breast cancer (67%) required more information than they actually received. Nevertheless, 17% of BACUP users were happy with the received information and did not require anything else, while 16% couldn't think of or didn't know what information they would have found useful at the time of diagnosis or at the time of survey questioning.

Additional information	(%)
Yes, they would have liked to receive more information	67
Could't think/didn't know what further information would be helpful	16
No, they did not require any additional information	17

Of those (67%) that required additional information, 37% would have liked information about support groups, and especially contact with other patients. 26% would have liked to know more about their cancer (types, causes, meaning, etc.). Treatment, emotional support, and written information were also among the commonest requests.

Specific useful information	(%)
Support groups (including patient-to-patient)	37
Breast cancer-specific information	26
Treatment (excluding prognosis and surgery)	18
Prognosis	12
Surgery	12
Emotional support/reassurance	19
Booklets/leaflets (not specified)	19
BACUP booklets/leaflets	9
Other	9

E) Comments

It can be seen from the above that most of the breast cancer patients *were treated well and received information at the time of the original diagnosis.* Most were told by a consultant surgeon in an appropriate place and they spent 15–29 minutes with him or her. A high proportion also received satisfactory information. Moreover, compared with a previous BACUP survey, patients seemed to be better informed and treated than other cancer patients.

Breast cancer patients quoted:
'The surgeon was quite concerned about the impact of the news on both me and my husband. He offered us a cup of tea before we left in order to help us collect our thoughts!'

'Everyone had been as helpful as they could be.'

'I have seen a breast care nurse since and I feel well informed and supported.'

'Very good service. If anything, too much information. However, I feel I was lucky to get referred to a breast cancer centre. I feel it was a bit of a lottery; fortunately I got the winning ticket.'

Nonetheless, *the given information was not sufficient* for the majority of patients (67%). It was mainly verbal, general information about the cancer and treatment options (70%) and in some cases booklets/leaflets (30%). Little information was given about counselling and support services.

What most people (67%) would have liked to receive was written information and contact details of support groups, more information about breast cancer, and information on treatment and emotional support.

People commented:
'Initially it was very difficult. I needed to be told this happens to lots of people and they get through it. It would have been helpful to have information on support groups and BACUP.'

'I wanted to know more details about what I had got, what was going to happen next, what the treatment might be.'

'I would have liked to have met someone who had had a mastectomy in outpatients. I would like to have been given information on what having cancer meant.'

'How I was going to cope with it? I felt as if I could have done with a bit of extra support somehow down the line.'

Written information appears to be preferable:
'I would like to be given information booklets. It brings it home to you that you are not the only one. You can read booklets again and again.'

'I would have liked to read some background information about the choices I was given, i.e. surgery and radiotherapy.'

Even if people were in 'shock' when they were given the diagnosis, they would request some additional information later on:

'I was in 'shock'. I didn't think about what would have been useful to ask. I would have needed to know about causes.'

'I was so shocked as I was expecting it not to be cancer. I am not sure what I wanted exactly at the moment. Telephone numbers of where to phone for information and support booklets/leaflets might be helpful.'

'I really needed something written. I would have welcomed some booklets and leaflets so that I could have read them afterwards when the shock had worn off.'

Despite the generally perceived good treatment of breast cancer patients, mistreatment and communication problems still exist:

'I felt let down because the specialist 'guaranteed' that the lump was not malignant—but then it turned out that it was.'

'I lost confidence in the breast care nurse immediately. When we were left alone, I asked her if there is anything that can be done. She said, 'there is no cure.'

'I felt unsupported after discharge. Delayed contact from health professionals—no communication.'

'I was treated like a number, insensitively handled when I was first told (mammogram, needle biopsy). However, later they were very good.'

The most extreme cases:

'The surgeon half turned away from me and said, "I'm sorry, it was malignant". I was not given any information. I got more support from other women in same situation.'

'It was a terrible experience. The surgeon who did the operation just came up to the bed in the ward with his understudies at visiting time. He said, "it was a nasty lump". I just flipped out, got dressed, and ran out of the hospital.'

'Nobody told me I had cancer. I was told that if I woke up after the operation and had a drip it would be bad news!'

Nonetheless, the way breast cancer patients are treated seems to be improving with time as health professionals and people in general become aware of different issues of breast cancer. A person that had a recurrence after 10 years felt the information and support was much better this time. However, as the above individuals' experience shows, information and treatment of cancer patients needs further improvement.

BACUP Cancer Information Service

April 1996/March 1997 Breast Cancer Enquiries (27.9% of the total 40 925 enquiries) Geographic (UK) distribution (excluding unknown location enquirers)

Region	(%)
North	3.7
Yorkshire	7.3
East Midlands	5.5
East Anglia	4.0
Greater London	15.6
South East (excluding London)	28.8
South West	10.5
West Midlands	7.8
North West	6.7
Scotland	5.7
Wales	3.2
Others	1.2
Total	100.0

April 1996/March 1997 Breast Cancer Enquiries (27.9% of the total 40 925 enquiries) Type of enquirer

Type of enquirer	(%)
Diagnosed patients	59.1
Friends/relatives of diagnosed patients	28.5
Undiagnosed persons/friends/relatives	6.6
Health professionals	2.4
Students	1.5
General public	0.7
Others/unspecified	1.0
Total	**100.0**

Note:

Friends/relatives of diagnosed patients include:	
Friends/relatives of diagnosed patients	28.0
Friends/relatives of deceased patients	0.5
Total	**28.5**
Undiagnosed persons/friends/relatives include:	
Undiagnosed persons	4.9
Friends/relatives of undiagnosed persons	1.7
Total	**6.6**
Health professionals include:	
Nurses	1.9
Other health professionals	0.5
Total	**2.4**
Others/unspecified include:	
Organisations/support groups	0.1
Other non-health professionals	0.5
Unknown	0.3
Total	**1.0**

April 1996/March 1997 Breast Cancer Enquiries. Relatives and friends of diagnosed patients only (28.5% of all breast enquirers). Subject of enquiry—groups

Subject of enquiry	(%)
Administrative	4.4
Publications	47.0
Previous/screen/risk factors	8.0
General treatment enquiries	26.7
Specific therapy enquiries	41.3
Site-specific information	35.4
Other medical enquiries	38.5
Emotional support	44.9
Support services	11.5
Other support enquiries	30.7

Nurses can code up to six subjects of enquiry for every enquirer.

The above percentages represent the number of relatives/friends of breast cancer patients who asked about one or more of the particular subjects belonging to the group, irrespective of whether other subjects were raised. For example, 47% of all relatives/friends (100%) requested publications, while 41.3% of all relatives/friends needed information for one or more specific therapies.

If group statistics are quoted, it is advisable to refer to subjects included in every group for clarification. See '*Subject of enquiry—analytical*'.

April 1996/March 1997 Breast Cancer Enquiries. Relatives and friends of diagnosed patients only (28.5% of all breast enquirers). Subject of enquiry—analytical

Subject of enquiry	(%)
Administrative enquiries	4.4
Publications	47.0
Prevention/screen/risk factors	
Breast screening	2.6
Cervical screening	0.0
Other screening	0.3
Risk factors	5.2
Warning symptoms	1.6

Subject of enquiry	(%)
Treatment enquiries	
General treatment	5.2
Treatment side-effects	15.3
Drugs queries	1.4
Research/clinical trials	4.0
Treatment centres/Drs	4.7
Specific therapy enquiries	
Auto/allo BMT and stem cell transplant	0.5
Chemotherapy	18.8
Complementary/alternative therapies	3.1
Hormonal therapy	12.0
Immunotherapy	0.2
Radiotherapy	16.6
Surgery	9.2
Other treatment	1.0
Site-specific information	**35.4**
Other medical enquiries	
Clarification of information received	13.9
Death and dying	2.8
Diagnostic procedure	2.3
Diet and nutrition	2.6
Follow-up	0.5
Pain control	3.1
Prognosis	12.7
Recurrence	5.2
Second opinion	1.6
Symptom control	4.2
Emotional support	
Bereavement	0.7
Emotional support/reassurance	41.6
Narratives/catharsis	2.6
Support services	
Community care	3.8
Counselling services	3.7
Support groups	5.4
Other support enquiries	
Health professional communications	11.7
Personal/family/friends communications	16.4
Sexuality/sexual problems	0.3
Complaint about health care received	1.7

Subject of enquiry	(%)
Financial concerns	3.7
Practical support	2.3
Other subject of enquiry	0.9

Risk factors include heredity/genetics (4.4%) and other.
Community care includes general, Macmillan enquiries, and other.
Practical support includes getting equipment and prostheses/wigs.
Financial concerns include general insurance, holiday/travel insurance, benefits, etc.

April 1996/March 1997 Breast Cancer Enquiries. Relatives and friends of diagnosed patients only (28.5% of all breast enquirers). Subject of enquiry—the commonest enquiries

The commonest enquiries	(%)
Publications	47.0
Emotional support	41.6
Site-specific information	35.4
Chemotherapy	18.8
Radiotherapy	16.6
Personal/family/friends communications	16.4
Treatment side-effects	15.3
Information clarification	13.9
Prognosis	12.7
Hormonal therapy	12.0
Health professional communication	11.7
Surgery	9.2
Support groups	5.4
Recurrence	5.2
General treatment	5.2
Risk factors	5.2
Treatment centres/Drs	4.7

Nurses can code up to six subjects of enquiry for every enquirer.
The percentages represent the proportion of relatives/friends of breast cancer patients who asked about a particular subject, irrespective of whether other subjects were raised. Therefore the total is not 100%.

April 1996/March 1997 Breast Cancer Enquiries. Diagnosed patients only (59.1% of all breast enquirers). Subject of enquiry—the commonest enquiries

The commonest enquiries	(%)
Emotional support	45.8
Publications	44.6
Site-specific information	32.0
Treatment side-effects	31.5
Chemotherapy	22.8
Hormonal therapy	20.7
Information clarification	17.5
Radiotherapy	15.6
Surgery	15.1
Health professional communication	12.9
Recurrence	9.6
Prognosis	6.1
Personal/family/friends communication	6.0
Symptom control	4.8

Nurses can code up to six subjects of enquiry for every enquirer.

The percentages represent the proportion of breast cancer patients who asked about a particular subject, irrespective of whether other subjects were raised. Therefore the total is not 100%.

April 1996/March 1997 Breast Cancer Enquiries. Diagnosed patients only (59.1% of all breast enquirers). Subject of enquiry—groups

Subject of enquiry	(%)
Administrative	1.9
Publications	44.6
Prevention/screen/risk factors	5.1
General treatment enquiries	37.9
Specific therapy enquiries	57.6
Site-specific information	32.0
Other medical enquiries	39.9
Emotional support	48.5
Support services	5.5
Other support enquiries	24.3

Nurses can code up to six subjects of enquiry for every enquirer.

The above percentages represent the number of breast cancer patients who asked about one or more of the particular subjects belonging to the group, no matter if other subjects were raised.

For example, 44.6% of all patients with breast cancer (100%) requested publications, while 57.6% of all patients needed information for one or more specific therapies.

If group statistics are quoted, it is advisable to refer to subjects included in every group for clarification. See *Subject of enquiry—analytical*.

April 1996/March 1997 Breast Cancer Enquiries. Diagnosed patients only (59.1% of all breast enquirers). Subject of enquiry—analytical

Subject of enquiry	(%)
Administrative enquiries	1.9
Publications	44.6
Prevention/screen/risk factors	
Breast screening	0.8
Cervical screening	0.2
Other screening	0.3
Risk factors	2.7
Warning symptoms	1.5

Subject of enquiry	(%)
Treatment enquiries	
General treatment	2.2
Treatment side-effects	31.5
Drugs queries	0.9
Research/clinical trials	2.8
Treatment centres/Drs	3.6
Specific therapy enquiries	
Auto/allo BMT and stem cell transplant	0.7
Chemotherapy	22.8
Complementary/alternative therapies	3.2
Hormonal therapy	20.7
Immunotherapy	0.1
Radiotherapy	15.6
Surgery	15.1
Other treatment	0.5
Site-specific information	32.0
Other medical enquiries	
Clarification of information received	17.5
Death and dying	0.5
Diagnostic procedure	3.6
Diet and nutrition	3.6
Follow-up	2.4
Pain control	2.3
Prognosis	6.1
Recurrence	9.6
Second opinion	2.1
Symptom control	4.8
Emotional support	
Bereavement	0.1
Emotional support/reassurance	45.8
Narratives/catharsis	2.4
Support services	
Community care	0.6
Counselling services	1.2
Support groups	4.0
Other support enquiries	
Health professional communications	12.9
Personal/family/friends communications	6.0
Sexuality/sexual problems	1.8
Complaint about health care received	1.9

Subject of enquiry	(%)
Financial concerns	4.2
Practical support	2.1
Other subject of enquiry	1.2

Risk factors include heredity/genetics (1%) and other.

Practical support includes getting equipment and prostheses/wigs.

Financial concerns include general insurance, holiday/travel insurance, benefits, mortgages etc.

Nurses can code up to six subjects of enquiry for every enquirer.

The percentages represent the proportion of breast cancer patients who asked about a particular subject, irrespective of whether other subjects were raised. Therefore the total is not 100%.

As outlined in some of the above studies, the majority of patients surveyed wished to participate in the decision-making process (Cassileth *et al.* 1980; Blanched *et al.* 1988; Degner and Russell 1988; Brandt 1991), while others preferred their clinicians to take the decisions (Ingelfinger 1980; Sutherland *et al.* 1989; Degner and Sloane 1992; Bilodeau and Degner 1996).

In summary, lack of information is often cited in patient satisfaction surveys as a significant complaint (Locker and Dunt 1978; Maslin 1994; Rothert *et al.* 1994). It has been suggested (Tyron and Leonard 1965; Greer 1979) that giving surgical patients information in advance results in an improved post-operative recovery. Richards *et al.* (1995) state:

'involving patients in the decision making process could have both advantages and disadvantages for them. Proponents of offering choice may hope that this will lead to higher levels of patient satisfaction with care, and improved acceptance of treatment. It might also lessen psychiatric morbidity and improve quality of life. Against this, offering choice could place an undue burden of responsibility on patients. Revealing uncertainty about 'best treatment' could lead to a loss of confidence in the doctor. Provision of complex information required to make a valid choice may lead to confusion and could challenge a psychological response of denial or avoidance. Choice of treatment which subsequently proves unsuccessful might induce feelings of self blame and regret in the patient'.

Studies addressing psychiatric morbidity in breast cancer patients have indicated that it is not necessarily the type of operation that is the sole cause of anxiety or depression. Fear of recurrence and death are high on the agenda for many women, and this will have an impact on the choice made (Fallowfield *et al*. 1986; 1990).

Not wishing to take an active decision about the final choice of treatment, as previously stated, may not necessarily mean a total lack of desire for information. Cassileth *et al*. (1980) make the point that only approximately 60% of patients expressed a preference to participate in decisions regarding medical care and treatment, compared with more than 95% who wanted detailed information. Sutherland *et al*. (1989) suggest the results of this study indicated that patients 'may actively seek information to satisfy an as yet unidentified aspect of psychological autonomy that does not necessarily include participation in decision making'. Fallowfield *et al*. (1986; 1990*a,b*) likewise found that a desire for well-communicated information may not necessarily lead to a patient wishing to take sole responsibility for treatment decisions.

Gray (1990) suggested that once the word 'cancer' is used, patients often do not hear the rest of the conversation. Patients can and do change their minds regarding their desire to access information over a period of time (Priestman 1986). Patients may experience many conflicting emotions, including numbness, disbelief, anger, fear, hope, and despair (Buckman 1986; Priestman 1986). This sequence of emotions can make information-giving generally, or decision-making specifically, difficult at the time of diagnosis. Many patients find it difficult to comprehend what is being said and many find it difficult to remember what they have been told (Watson *et al*. 1988; Hogbin and Fallowfield 1989; Maslin 1993).

Goldie (1982, p. 132) pointed out that often staff, by putting themselves in the shoes of their patients, misunderstand the patients' actual thoughts and feelings. As a result, staff feel they already know a patient's view and therefore do not give the patient the opportunity to express their own opinion. Goldie also stated 'Sometimes the hospital, or part of it, can become like a totalitarian state, with a limitation on the subject's freedom to think and act independently'.

Reynolds *et al*. (1981, p. 227) suggest that 'physicians and nursing staff see a woman as a patient, a person and a statistic, the patient often has a difficult time understanding what is happening to her and why'. The patient may wonder what is uppermost in the clinician's mind when treatment options are suggested. They go on to suggest that information is generally lacking for patients and their families—no matter how good a job the physician and hospital staff are doing in trying to communicate important information (Maslin 1994). For some patients, information gathering becomes a coping mechanism. Information for this group of people enables them to have some control over their disease and its treatment. Information supplies them with options and options may lead to encouraging possibilities (Kfir and Slevin 1991).

Fallowfield *et al.* (1994*b*, p. 203), discussing their 1990 study, stated 'One of the primary findings was that although there were fewer cases of anxiety and depression in the group of women treated by surgeons who offered 'choice' wherever possible, choice was not the determining factor. Consulting style, in particular offering satisfactory information about treatment options, was crucial to long-term adjustment.' Fallowfield *et al.* (1994*a*, p. 448), reporting three-year follow-up data of their 1990 study (Fallowfield *et al.* 1990*b*), stated

'23 of the 62 women who were offered choice found it difficult to make a decision; eight refused to choose. Women were asked how they felt about having been asked to choose their operation. Twenty six expressed positive reactions, 13 were unable to say, and 10 were unenthusiastic. Five women, four of whom had chosen breast conservation, expressed doubts about their original decision; two eventually underwent mastectomy, one because of recurrence of the cancer and the other because severe problems after radiotherapy. The remaining 48 patients, nine of whom subsequently developed recurrence, did not regret their choice.'

Fallowfield *et al.* (1994*b*, p. 206) concluded:

'Women with breast cancer seem to benefit form the provision of clear information about treatment and, if appropriate, reasons why the doctor would recommend one treatment over another. If suitable, understandable information is provided, time to think and maybe to discuss the implications either with the doctor or an adequately trained specialist nurse, then an offer to take part in decision making if women so wish may significantly affect good adjustment.'

5

Approaches to shared decision-making

A.M. Maslin

The evidence appears to support the case for a sentient adult women with breast cancer having a right to express her autonomy, if she so wishes, by accessing accurate evidence-based information relating to her disease and treatment options, and that this information should be communicated effectively to her. But how can a woman with breast cancer access the information and participate, again if she so wishes, in the shared decision-making process? This chapter reviews the common, and a selection of the less common, methods available for the sharing information with patients.

Person-to-person verbal information

It is widely recognized that communication is one of the most important aspects of patient care (Fallowfield *et al.* 1986; 1987; 1990*a,b*; 1994*a,b*; Maguire *et al.* 1980; 1983; 1986; Maguire and Faulkner 1988*b,c*; 1990; Roberts 1990), and is an area of considerable dissatisfaction as revealed by surveys of patient experience (Cartwright 1964; Rapheal 1969; Parkin 1976; Reynolds 1978; Buckman 1986; Priestman 1986; Blum and Blum 1991). Ley (1988) reported a median dissatisfaction rate with medical communication of 38%. Blum and Blum (1991) demonstrated similar findings in their study looking at patient-team communications. They found 25% of callers to a community-based agency identified patient-physician communications as their primary concern. Fallowfield and Baum (1989) stated

'We have important data emerging from studies suggesting that the way in which the surgeon conducts the 'bad news' consultation, i.e. informing the patient of the diagnosis and treatment options, can have a major impact on short and long term psychological outcome'.

Fallowfield and Baum (1989) argued strongly that the 'bad news interviews' were crucial in the patient/clinician relationship and that an appropriately trained nurse counsellor in partnership with a department of psychological medicine could also facilitate a reduction in a breast cancer patient's psychiatric morbidity (Maguire *et al.* 1978; 1982; Watson *et al.* 1988).

Problems arising from poor communication are not solely confined to the medical profession. Macleod (1982) and Wilkinson (1992) likewise demonstrated that nurses often engage in brief, infrequent communication interactions which are often task orientated. If there is dissatisfaction with communication and the exchange of information, how can any patient give informed consent? Hughes (1993) conducted a study examining the relationship between information about breast cancer treatment options and patients' choices of treatment. The group studied consisted of women facing either a wide local excision followed by radiotherapy or a mastectomy. The amount of information provided for each patient was recorded on an observer check list. The information was primarily shared verbally. Follow-up telephone calls were conducted 6–8 weeks after the surgery. Hughes states

'The results indicate that subjects' choice of treatment was unrelated to the amount of information they received during their clinic visit. Manner of presentation also did not influence treatment selection. However, treatment selection was related to the amount of information they received prior to their clinic visit ($p < 0.01$). The results also indicate that patients' recall of information about treatments and associated risks is exceedingly poor.'

Almost 50% of the women who chose wide local excision could not recall characteristics of their treatment and associated risks, and this rose to 66% in the mastectomy group. This finding is of obvious importance when considering the information given at the time of diagnosis. Another interesting finding was that women who opted for a mastectomy received significantly more information about their operation and breast cancer treatment prior to their clinic visits from informal sources like friends and family (Hughes 1993). It is obvious that this information may or may not be accurate, and this needs to be borne in mind by health care professionals.

Replying to Apolone and colleagues in the *BMJ* (Fallowfield *et al.* 1990*b*), Fallowfield confirmed that:

'Women treated by surgeons who offered 'choice' whenever possible fared better in terms of psychiatric morbidity than women in other surgeon groups. This was true even when women could not be permitted choice for technical reasons. This implies that those surgeons who were prepared to allow women to participate in the decision-making process whenever possible differed in some qualitative way from those who tended to make the treatment decision for their patients. We could suggest that the surgeons who offered choice were perhaps more skilled in the art of communication, including the provision of good information and psychological support.'

The evidence clearly shows that verbal information effectively communicated to a patient with breast cancer can have a significant impact on patient satisfaction and the ability to adjust to diagnosis and treatment. Difficulties with communicating information verbally involve, on the part of the professional, at times, lack of knowledge, lack of expertise, and lack of time and on the part of the patient, at times, a lack of general understanding or an inability to understand due to the impact of stress and selective perception (Greer 1979; Watson *et al.* 1984; Greer *et al.* 1990).

Use of literature

Ellis *et al.* (1986) demonstrated that the addition of written information to the provision of verbal information improved patient understanding and recall. Webb (1987) discussed the range of topics and the variety of ways written information is available to patients within the cancer setting. Webb expresses the view that good-quality written material with appropriate illustrations can be a powerful medium for facilitating patient education and understanding. Webb states 'a permanent record or hard copy of factual information allows reinforcement of material when the patient and family want it'. One problem with the written word is that often the level of literacy required by the reader is too high, although its effectiveness may be enhanced if it is prepared with the reading age of the user specifically in mind (Meade *et al.* 1994).

Luker and Caress (1989) pointed out that nurses are rarely trained in the 'breadth and depth of knowledge necessary to teach patients who, by view of their illness, may have special learning difficulties'. Maslin *et al.* (1993) noted that in a sample of 200 patients at high risk of developing breast cancer or a confirmed diagnosis of breast cancer, 75% received or remember receiving written material on entering a clinical trial, and 99% of that group claim to have read it. When this same sample of patients expressed written comments on the information they received they wanted access to more explicit information, particularly in relation to side-effects of treatments and drugs.

Chapman *et al.* (1995) reported a study which examined the effect of providing breast cancer information on patients, and the effect of providing information on treatment options on the individual's choice of treatment. They used undergraduate students as surrogate patients and assessed their baseline knowledge on the disease and its treatment options. They also ascertained the individuals' initial preferences for treatment, from wide local excision followed by radiotherapy, mastectomy followed by reconstruction, to a mastectomy followed by use of a breast prosthesis. This was done both prior to and after reading a booklet or watching an interactive videotape of the relevant information. Treatment choices were not affected by reading the booklet but a preference shift was noted, after watching the videotape, towards breast-conserving surgery. This study is a useful indicator, but the use of surrogate patients makes the reliability of its findings in relation to breast cancer patients difficult to ascertain.

One difficulty with literature is that it caters for a group of patients and is not always able to meet the needs of patients who are outside the norm. For example, hospital literature aimed at women with breast cancer may take general examples and scenarios, but may not be able to meet the needs of a patient with a rarer condition, i.e. inflammatory breast cancer or Paget's disease. Another difficulty with written information obtained in a library or straight off the internet is that it may not be directly applicable to the patient and therefore the opposite problem is experienced, where the patient accesses copious information, some of which may not be relevant. In view of this, it may be useful to adopt information-sharing methods which are tailored to the patient (Hogbin and Fallowfield 1989), e.g. the use of audiotapes.

Use of tape recorders

Use of tape recorders for reinforcement of information on hernia repair was used by Baskerville *et al.* (1985). They aimed to give and record appropriate information in a relaxed setting with the patients, and then provided the patients with a copy of the recording to take home. Baskerville *et al.* (1985) reported 90% of the patients found the tape recording adequate and accurate. They noted that the voice of the surgeon appeared to give the audio recording a greater sense of authority than written material.

Hogbin and Fallowfield (1989) studied the effectiveness of using a tape recorder during cancer patients' 'bad news' interviews. In total they gave 46 patients audio recordings of their interview with the clinician when the 'bad news' and possible treatment options were discussed. The authors aimed to discover (a) whether it was practical to record the consultation in an ordinary outpatient department, (b) what differences, if any, this made to the consultation and the way information was communicated, and (c) how useful this process was to the cancer patients. Of the 46 patients 39 listened to the tape recording and of that 39, 38 listened to it with a friend or relative. All 39 patients found the tape recording helpful and 15 stated that it contained information they had forgotten. Of the 39 patients, eight felt that the tape, or part of it, upset them, but 31 said it did not.

Hogbin and Fallowfield (1989, p. 332) use a number of patient quotes to illustrate the usefulness of the tapes; these included:

'The tape was a wonderful idea. I was able to play it several times to my very large family.'

'This (the tape) was a tremendous help as it is impossible to recall everything said when one is in a state of shock.'

Knowles (1992) reported a randomized study of 34 patients with advanced cancer, half of whom were randomized to have their consultation tape recorded. Their aim was to see if the use of an audiotape increased information retention and reduced anxiety and depression levels. This study was small and therefore the results were only indicators. Patients who had the tape recording appeared to show a decrease in their mean anxiety scores after 1 week from 7.1 to 3.1 (HAD, Zigmond and Snaith 1983) and a substantial increase in information recall at a second interview. The control group, however, showed only a marginal improvement in information recall and retained a mean anxiety score of 6.1. Patients did, however, express largely positive feelings and confirmed the view that the tapes were helpful, not only for the patient but the immediate and extended family.

The use of audiotapes would appear, on balance, to elicit a largely favourable response and helps to address issues relating to the stress a patient experiences, which may affect their ability to hear and understand a diagnosis or treatment options, particularly during a 'bad news' interview.

Use of videos

A variety of linear videos have been made. Videotapes have been found to be as effective as other forms of instruction and more effective than printed materials alone (Gagliano 1988; Uzark *et al.* 1985; Neilson and Sheppard 1988; Tongue 1991). Uzark *et al.* (1985) found the use of videos for parents of children with congenital heart defects resulted in improved parental understanding, and as a result, the families were more willing to comply with recommendations for care.

Meade *et al.* (1994) compared the effectiveness of written information and videotaped information on patients with limited literacy who had a diagnosis of cancer of the colon. The results showed an increase in knowledge and understanding in each group but only short-term memory recall was evaluated. The authors suggested that because the literature was prepared specifically to meet the needs of people with limited literacy, this may have made the literature more effective than the videotapes.

Tongue (1991) conducted a study of a video-based information system (VISP), for general practice waiting room areas, to assess its value to patients. He found that it was possible to produce a low-cost information system for patient waiting areas, but found staff and patients expressed a variety of views as to what it would be most helpful for the system to concentrate on. Tongue felt health promotion material merited consideration. Webb (1987) suggested the time cancer patients spent in outpatients could be used effectively by the introduction of self-directed educational programmes. Videos currently available on breast cancer treatment options vary between those specifically designed for the patient and those developed as a teaching tool for professionals, e.g. Cleese *et al.* 'Breast Cancer' (1993). These videos have not been subject to evaluation in a clinical trial. If an individual patient has access to or the ability to purchase a video, they can see material which is not specifically prepared for them.

Videos are useful in countries like the UK where access to a video recorder is fairly commonplace. The videos can be borrowed at little cost and the patient can view the material in the surroundings of their choice. Difficulties may arise if the patient has questions which cannot be answered immediately or if the material, although accurate, is not appropriate to their own situation, for example treatments may be discussed which are not an appropriate option for the individual.

Use of computers

Computer assisted learning (CAL) for patients is a new but rapidly developing field. CAL does appear to be helpful in patient education (Fisher *et al.* 1977; Deardorff 1986). As far back as 1977 Fisher *et al.* demonstrated that even the elderly found the technology acceptable. Deardoff (1986) found that CAL was rated more highly than the written material. An important feature of CAL is that the patient is free to cover the material in their own time, to repeat the information, and in many cases to do this without the fear of taking up too much of the professionals' time (Deardoff 1986). With the availability of CD and laser disc systems the information can be given verbally as well as visually, which is helpful to those who are deaf or blind. The use of touch control screens enables those unfamiliar with keyboards to use the systems rapidly. Luker and Caress (1989, p. 716) rightly state that the usefulness of these systems is largely dependent on the quality of the software in interaction with the user.

Comprehensive Health Enhancement Support System (CHESS)

CHESS was developed as a user-friendly interactive computer-based system designed to provide information and support to women facing a breast cancer diagnosis. This system was developed by a group at the University of Wisconsin, Madison, and has been piloted (Gustafson *et al.* 1993; McTavish *et al.* 1993). The system will soon be available for general use (Mort *et al.* 1995). The 'services include answers to common questions, a database of articles and brochures, a tutorial that explains social services ... personal stories, and an on-line discussion group' (Mort *et al.* 1995, p. 7).

Bedside decision board for adjuvant therapy decisions

This is a tool which was developed in Ontario to help ascertain patients' preferences for adjuvant chemotherapy (Levine *et al.* 1992). The tool is a decision board which provides patients with probabilities of recurrence and quality-of-life outcomes associated with chemotherapy. The aim of Levine *et al.*'s study was to develop an instrument to help clinicians inform patients with breast cancer of the risk and benefits of adjuvant chemotherapy as demonstrated by clinical trials, and help them decide whether to accept or reject a treatment option. A pilot was conducted among healthy volunteers to determine their preferences and to assess for reliability and validity. Although this was useful, it is known that surrogate patients' and control patients' views do frequently differ from those of patients directly involved (Slevin *et al.* 1988; Maslin 1993). The decision board was been found to be acceptable and helpful to 37 newly presenting, high-risk patients with node negative breast cancer (Levine *et al.* 1992).

The shared decision-making program (SDP)/interactive video disc system (IVD)

McNeil *et al.* (1982) stated:

'there is a growing appreciation in the general public and medical profession of the need to incorporate patient preferences into medical decision making. To achieve this goal, the physician must provide the patient with the data about possible outcomes of the available therapies and the patient must be able to comprehend and use the data.'

In a 1991 American Medical Association survey 69% of the respondents claimed they were losing faith in doctors and only

42% said their doctor adequately explains disease and treatment (Willson 1992). This is not surprising given that it is estimated that by the American National Board of Medical Practitioners that doctors, on average, spend less than seven minutes talking to patients and this figure has fallen from 11 in 1975 (Willson 1992).

Mort (1996) drew attention to the fact that in some instances (Mort quoted hormone replacement therapy (HRT) as an example) there was widespread variation in prescribing patterns. Mort acknowledges that there will be some expected variation, but what was unexpected was the variation in prescribing which appeared to be systematic and linked to geographic region, physician gender, and other non-clinical factors. With this known variation it is reasonable that some patients may wish to know why there is a variation in practice and may wish to participate in the decision to evaluate what therapy, if any, is offered.

Mulley (1990) hypothesized that active efforts to involve patients in decisions made about their care should improve outcomes by better matching treatments with patient values and needs. In an attempt to address this quantity and quality issue with regard to the patients' access to information, the Foundation for Informed Medical Decision-Making, a non-profit foundation, developed and produced four initial interactive multimedia programmes (Mulley 1990; 1992; Kasper *et al.* 1992*a*,*b*; Wennberg 1992*b*,*c*; Wagner *et al.* 1993) dealing with benign prostate disease, hypertension, lower back pain, and early breast cancer. These aimed to allow individual patients to explore the details of the conditions.

The programmes are a mixture of documentary-style video clips, still shots, diagrams, and text. The programs are ported to a DOS-based playback system, a Dell 486 equipped with a Sony GVM 1315 TS touch screen, and a Sony LDP 1450 video disc player. To create the programmes the developers consulted with doctors and patient focus groups to ascertain the questions that are important to patients.

The interactive video disc (IVD) shared decision-making program (SDP)

'is a video program presented in an interactive format using an video disc player, a modified microcomputer, a video monitor, and a printer.

It is designed for use in the health care provider setting. Information about a given medical condition is provided along with descriptions of the benefits and harms associated with the relevant treatment alternatives' (Kasper *et al.* 1992*a*).

Barry *et al.* (1995) conducted a study to evaluate an IVD/SDP for men with benign prostate disease. The study was a prospective cohort study conducted in three hospital-based urology clinics. Data from 373 men were suitable for analysis. The patients rated the programme for length, clarity, balance, and value of the programme. 77% of the patients were very positive and 16% were generally positive about the programme's usefulness. Patients rated the programme as generally clear, informative, and balanced. The results suggested that patients can be helped to participate in treatment decisions, and support a randomized trial of the shared decision-making programme.

The King's Fund Centre for Development (England) has supported pilot studies looking at the system's usefulness for patients. Data are available for patients with benign prostate disease, hypertension, and breast cancer (Shepherd *et al.* 1995; Maslin *et al.* 1998).

Shepherd *et al.* (1995) conducted a descriptive cohort study piloting interactive videos in general practices to help inform patients regarding treatment choices for mild hypertension and benign prostatic hypertrophy. Fifty-four patients with mild hypertension and 29 with benign prostatic hypertrophy were recruited from eight general practices in Oxfordshire. The patients' views of the video, treatment preference, level of involvement in treatment decision, and satisfaction with the decision-making process were assessed, as well as the GP's view on subsequent consultations. The patients and GPs were favourable in their responses, with 71% of patients saying it definitely helped with their treatment decision and GPs indicated in 82% of cases that they found the IVD helpful. The results of this study provided support for the view that a randomized controlled study was needed to evaluate the impact of the IVD on the doctor–patient relationship, on subsequent treatment decisions, on health outcomes and patient well being.

Naylor (1995), when discussing evidence-based medicine (EBM) pointed out that EBM 'offers little help in many grey zones of practice where the evidence about risk benefit ratios of competing clinical options is incomplete or contradictory'. The aim of an IVD system is to facilitate shared decision-making in these grey areas, for those patients who would want it, by providing a computerized database of established, evidence-based 'knowledge' which will help to meet the information needs of patients and allow them to become involved in the decision-making process (Kasper *et al.* 1992). The patient's participation and value system are integral to the operation of the system.

Kasper *et al.* (1992*b*, p. 183) suggest:

'The shared decision and the process by which it is reached offer the best hope for improving patient satisfaction, increasing feelings of professionalism among providers, and promoting treatment choice on the basis of patient's values.'

De Vahl Davis (1992) states:

'informed consent implies that the information given has been received and understood, that it will be given without bias, and that the patient will have a real choice, whether it is to treat or not to treat, whether it is this treatment or that which should be used, whether to have an operation or not.'

The interactive video disc system, it is claimed, offers a unique opportunity to attempt to provide information with limited bias and to provide real choice.

Mort (1996) states that the IVD/SDM program

'is not designed to replace the physician in the decision making process. On the contrary, it complements the traditional physician/patient encounter. In practice, physicians identify eligible patients and advise them to use the programme.'

She points out that the information received assists some patients by giving them a working vocabulary which facilitates their encounters with their physicians, enabling more productive consultations.

The breast cancer SDP/IVD

A poorly informed breast cancer patient is more likely to be an anxious patient (Fallowfield *et al.* 1986). In the study looking at 101 breast cancer patients who had been randomized to either mastectomy or breast conservation, they were asked about the adequacy of the information they received from their doctors. Over half the patients were not satisfied with the information they received. As previously discussed, Maslin (1993) surveyed breast cancer patients' satisfaction with their experience when giving consent to join a clinical trial, especially in relation to information and support. Over 90% of the patients surveyed wanted access to specific written and verbal information, including risks/benefits and a comprehensive account of known side-effects.

Hack *et al.* (1994, p. 279) summed up the situation stating

'To enable cancer patients to contribute to the process of selecting their treatments, it may be necessary for them to have a sufficient amount of illness-treatment related knowledge. For example if women with T1 N0 M0 breast tumours are to choose between a modified radical mastectomy and breast conserving surgery, they may require information about the probability of success and side effects associated with each treatment alternative.'

There are a number of useful ways to provide information to patients, but how can we provide information to those breast cancer patients who wish it which is accurate, empathetic, unique to them, and consistent?

The interactive system provides research-based information on local and systemic treatment and also explores areas of uncertainty and variations in practice. The breast cancer IVD/SDP provides the patient with research-based evidence that is directly applicable to their own situation. They are able in the adjuvant therapy section to access general information about a hypothetical patient's risks of recurrence and mortality, but they are also able to access their own personal risks of recurrence and mortality figures. The patient is advised that this information may not apply in their case; it reflects the statistics which apply to a group of individuals in their situation. The information is presented verbally, visually, and diagramatically and includes figures for relative risk reduction, absolute risk reduction, difference in event-free survival, and the number of patients needed to be treated to achieve benefit.

One of the first available shared decision-making programs (SDP) for patients with cancer was produced in 1994 and was aimed at women with early breast cancer (Kasper *et al.* 1992;

Maslin *et al.* 1998). The programme summarized treatment options, with results for each option based on efficacy. The information available to the patient as indicated above includes odds for relapse and survival.

Maslin *et al.* (1998) piloted and evaluated the 'shared decision-making programme (SDP) for women with early breast cancer, looking at surgical and adjuvant treatment options using a personalized, computerized interactive laser disc system (IVD)'.

As previously stated the anxiety and depression found in women with early breast cancer can be reduced if they are seen by a clinician who communicates effectively with them and who aims to incorporate patient choice into treatment decisions, if this is possible and if the patient wishes (Fallowfield *et al.* 1990*a,b*). Women receiving treatment for breast cancer constitute a patient group in whom some of the questions surrounding communication choice and shared decision-making have been explored (Fallowfield *et al.* 1990*a,b*; Thornton 1992; Maslin 1993; 1994; Beaver *et al.* 1996). This study aimed to address some of the issues relating to shared decision-making in those areas where a choice of treatment option involves some degree of risk/benefit analysis.

The study aimed to pilot and evaluate the usefulness of a shared decision-making program for women with early breast cancer, looking at surgical and adjuvant treatment options using a personalized, computerized interactive laser disc system (Kasper *et al.* 1992*a,b*). The SDP/IVD aimed to provide the patient with information in areas where there is a genuine, but difficult, treatment option choice.

Specifically

1. To determine the acceptability of an IVD system, in addition to the standard informational care and support provided by the clinicians and clinical nurse specialist, as a means of providing information about the risks and benefits of treatment choices—surgery and subsequent adjuvant chemotherapy—for women with early breast cancer who are facing choices about treating their breast disease.

2. To determine whether providing information to women with early breast cancer using an interactive system significantly

reduces anxiety and depression associated with the diagnosis and treatment of this condition.

3. To determine whether providing information using an IVD system to women about treatment choices significantly increases patient satisfaction with the choice they have made.

The IVD/SDP system provided research-based information on local and systemic treatment for early breast cancer and also explored areas of uncertainty and variations in practice. The breast cancer IVD provided the patient with research-based evidence which is directly applicable to their own situation on both surgical and adjuvant treatment options. They were able in the adjuvant therapy section to access general information about a hypothetical patient's risks of recurrence and mortality, but they were also able to access their own personal risks of recurrence and mortality figures. The patient was advised that this information may not apply in their case. The information seen by the patient reflected the statistics which would apply to a group of individuals in their situation. The information was presented verbally, visually, and diagramatically and included figures for relative risk reduction, absolute risk reduction, difference in event-free survival, and the number needed to be treated to achieve benefit.

As stated above, the first available SDP for patients with cancer was produced in 1994 and was aimed at women with early breast cancer (Kasper *et al.* 1992*a,b*). The program summarizes treatment options with results for each option based on efficacy. The results, as indicated above, include odds for relapse and survival.

The interactive component to the system in the breast cancer IVD is expressed in two ways:

1. The patient's own details, e.g. age, tumour size, lymph node status, define the content of the first part of the IVD.
2. The patient is able to interact with the system by agreeing to proceed, have a break, or stop. In the second part of the system a 'learn more' section is available and the patient is able to interact with the content of this section at will, e.g. choosing material to watch, going over previous material, accessing new material, etc.

The IVD is different to a standard linear videotape in that it provides information which is unique to each patient, being tailored according to the personal details which are keyed in. The interactivity means patients can go forwards or backwards in the system. They can review material or they can opt out if they wish. The system also has programmed pauses to allow patients to take a break if required.

The breast cancer IVD database aims to:

1. Provide information on the management of individual patients with early breast cancer based on the current overview of randomized controlled trials.

2. Provide information on current areas of debate concerning the management of breast cancer and a rationale for treatments on offer.

3. Address issues relating to benefits and disadvantages of treatments based on the impact of a treatment on quality of life balanced against the possibility of extending life expectancy.

4. Address areas of current controversy and uncertainty.

5. Recognize that individual patients will have legitimate personal views, values, and preferences which may influence their choice of local or systemic treatment.

Mort *et al.* (1995, p. 5) state

'When women with early stage breast cancer who are suitable candidates for either surgical option (wide local excision followed by radiotherapy or mastectomy $\pm$ reconstruction) learn that their survival outcome is the same in either case, a broad range of outcomes become important to consider . . . Although many physicians and patients would agree that the most important outcome for women with early-stage breast cancer is survival, it is less likely that physicians and patients would agree in the relative importance of outcomes that relate more to the patient's quality of life. One woman may feel strongly that conserving the physical appearance or sensation of her breast is extremely important. Another woman may feel that removing the involved breast and reducing her chance of dealing with an in-breast ipsilateral recurrence and subsequent mastectomy is more important than conserving her breast. It bears emphasising that having a choice is not the same as having to make a decision.'

After using the interactive video system and standard informational care from their clinicians and clinical nurse specialist, the patient should (Mort *et al.* 1995)

1. Be able to make an informed treatment choice.
2. Have a rationale for their chosen treatment.
3. Understand the benefits, trade-offs, and impact on quality of life which may occur as a result of their choice.
4. Be in possession of a hard copy of the information they have accessed which is personalized.

An experimental, randomized study design was chosen to attempt to eliminate bias in apportioning the novel component, the IVD system. Patients, $n = 100$, were recruited from a specialist multidisciplinary breast unit. The women were recruited from the breast unit on the basis of a confirmed diagnosis of breast cancer, either by fine needle aspiration cytology or biopsy. The women all had a small localized primary breast cancer with no evidence of metastatic disease. When patients were recruited they were fully informed of the study prior to giving written consent and being randomized to either standard informational care with the full support of the multidisciplinary team or to the experimental group who, in addition to the full support of the multidisciplinary team, were offered use of the IVD to aid them in decision-making if they so wished (Fig. 5.1). Patients completed questionnaires at the time of recruitment and then again at 9 months post diagnosis.

The main outcome measures used were:

(a) Acceptability of the IVD.
   This was assessed using a simple Likert (Burns and Grove 1987) questionnaire asking the patient's opinion about the information content of the interactive videos, how it was presented, and what impact they felt it made on their decision about what treatments to choose.
(b) Assessment of health status.
   The SF36—a multidimensional health status profile—to measure changes in health status.

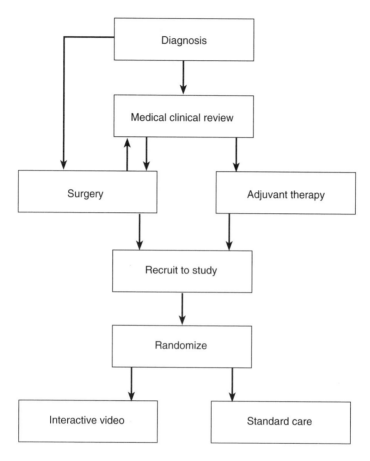

Fig. 5.1 Patients randomized at the time of surgical choice also have the opportunity to view the adjuvant video, where appropriate.

The choice of this questionnaire was based on:

(i) its ability to measure a wide number of variables including physical mobility, emotional well-being, social life, and overall well-being;
(ii) ease of use for patients. The version used is the Short Form 36 which has been developed from the much longer original (Brazier *et al.* 1992) with 36 questions covering eight dimensions;

(iii) its reliability and validity (McHorney *et al.* 1992; 1993);

(iv) the information that it was anticipated would be used by other groups evaluating other IVD programs from the Shared Decision Making Foundation, thus enabling some cross-comparison of data and;

(v) the fact that normative data exists to enable useful interpretation.

With 100 patients in the study it was possible to reliably detect a difference in the changes of these scores between the two groups of 0.6s where 's' is the standard deviation of the change within each patient. This difference can be detected with a probability of 85%.

If attention is focused on the percentage of patients who experience a fall with respect to their pretreatment value, then it will be possible (with 85% probability) to detect differences between the groups in the percentage showing a fall in the order of 35% v 10% or 50% v 20%.

(c) The Hospital Anxiety and Depression (HAD) scale (Zigmond and Snaith 1983).

This is a self assessment scale for the detection of anxiety and depressive states in a medical outpatient clinic (Bowling 1991) developed by Zigmond and Snaith (1983). It is a brief assessment of anxiety and depression, in which the patient rates each item on a four-point scale. Items relating to both emotional and physical disorder, e.g. headaches, are excluded so that items included are restricted to those based on the psychic symptoms of neurosis (Bowling 1991).

Items on the scale are scored from 0–3 to 3–0 depending on which way the question is worded. High scores indicate the presence of a problem. HAD depression scores of 7 or less are considered to be of no consequence, scores of 8–10 could indicate the possibility of anxiety or depression, and scores of 11 or more indicate a definite problem (Bowling 1991).

After nine months all the patients were asked to complete three questionnaires but at this point, in addition to the HAD and SF36, the third questionnaire aimed to elicit the patient's satisfaction with their treatment choice at nine months post diagnosis. Patients in the control group were asked to complete their initial questionnaires at the time they made their treatment decision and again, as outlined above, after nine months.

The exclusion criteria included:

- women who were pregnant
- women with clinical or mammographic evidence of bilateral breast cancer
- women with clinical or mammographic evidence of multicentric breast cancer (including gross multifocal disease or diffuse microcalcifications by mammography)
- women with a large tumour in relation to the size of the breast
- women with histopathological findings after biopsy of Paget's disease or inflammatory breast cancer
- women with tumours fixed to the chest wall
- women in whom the tumour was ulcerated
- women whose axillary lymph nodes were fixed and/or matted
- women with supraclavicular lymph nodes
- women with a chest X-ray indicative of lung metastases
- women with liver function tests suggestive of metastases
- women who, on physical examination, were found to have hepatomegaly
- women who had evidence of bone metastases as a result of a bone scan
- women in whom there is other clinical or diagnostic evidence of metastases
- women whose overall health would make mastectomy too life threatening to be an appropriate alternative
- women who had an absolute contraindication to radiotherapy
- women with severe hearing, vision, or cognitive impairment
- women who did not understand English.

One hundred patients were recruited over a two-year period. Fifty one women were randomized to see the IVD and 49 to standard care.

The comprehensive exclusion criteria were necessary to ensure that only patients with a genuine treatment choice were included in the study. Six patients were lost to follow-up. The women's ages ranged from 28 to 73 years with a mean of 52.1 years, with an even distribution between pre- and postmenopausal women.

At nine months 94% of questionnaires were returned, which was an excellent result for follow-up by postal questionnaire (Burns and Grove 1987).

The Hospital Anxiety and Depression scale overall summary scores for both groups indicated a significant fall in anxiety at 9 months ($p < 0.001$). There was no real change in the depression scores in either group, which were low at the start when compared with a normal age-matched population.

The SF36 general health questionnaire score indicated evidence of a slight fall overall, which was not significant. The scores for physical functioning indicated that there was an overall fall in the median score from 90 to 85 ($p = 0.01$). Likewise, in physical role functioning, there appears to be evidence of a fall overall, the median score falling from 100 to 50 ($p = 0.04$) at nine months. The mental health scores suggest a significant improvement in the IVD group, the median score rising from 60 at the outset to 68 at nine months ($p = 0.02$). However, the median score was 68 both pretreatment and at nine months in the standard care group. The scores for emotional role functioning also indicated an improvement overall at nine months.

The women's treatment option choices showed no statistically significant difference ($p = 0.08$) (Mann-Whitney U Test, Burns and Grove 1987, p. 494) (Fig. 5.2).

Opinions of the IVD: Of the patients who viewed the interactive videos (IVD) ($n = 51$), 82% found it just about right in length. Of those patients, 96% found the IVD interesting or very interesting. The majority of the participants, 92%, found it easy/very easy to understand. 72% felt they now had a much clearer idea about breast cancer. Of the viewers, 67% were 'Glad they had used the video and would use it again', but 28% stated they 'Found it helpful but would not necessarily use it again'. Overall, 94% felt they benefited from using the IVD. When asked if the patient would recommend the IVD to someone they knew with a diagnosis of breast cancer, 92% said 'yes' (see Figs 5.3–5.8).

Patients gave a mixed response when asked if the IVD had actually helped or influenced their decision. Just over half the

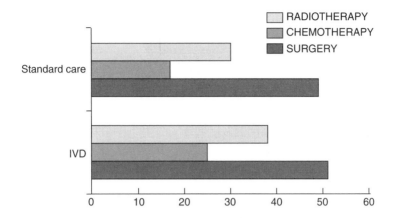

Fig. 5.2 Numbers of women recruited who chose surgery, chemotherapy, and/or radiotherapy.

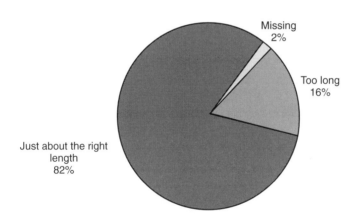

Fig. 5.3 Response to Interactive Video—length.

patients, 54%, stated that the IVD had been interesting but had not influenced their ultimate decision, but, 30% felt the IVD had definitely influenced their treatment decision. When asked if they had found any of the information worrying, 62% said they did not.

Views on the decision taken at nine months post diagnosis: Of the patients who were asked if the IVD for surgical treatment

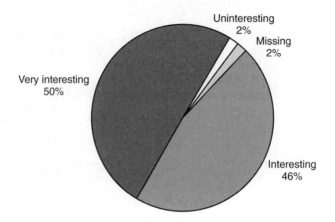

Fig. 5.4 Response to Interactive Video—response.

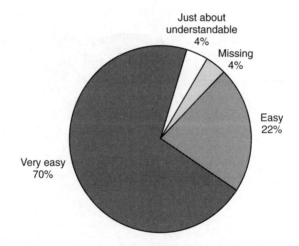

Fig. 5.5 Response to Interactive Video—understanding.

options changed their surgical treatment choice, only 12.5% indicated that it had. Of the patients who were asked if the IVD for adjuvant therapy changed the choice they ultimately made, 14.2% stated it had. The majority, 85%, said the IVD had not changed their adjuvant therapy choice.

The overall majority of patients, 81%, in both arms of the study stated quite clearly that the clinician was involved in

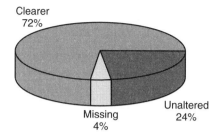

Fig. 5.6 Response to Interactive Video—knowledge.

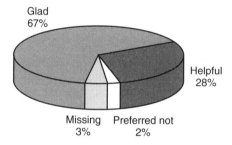

Fig. 5.7 Response to Interactive Video—appreciation.

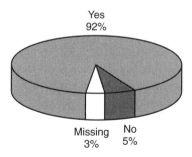

Fig. 5.8 Response to Interactive Video—recommendation.

making the treatment decision either by taking the decision on his own (21%), sharing the decision with the patient (16%), or sharing the decision with the patient and the breast care nurse (44%). The breast care nurse featured strongly in the decision-making process. Only 10 patients, 11%, stated that they alone made the decision on the choice of treatment option (Figs 5.9–5.10). When

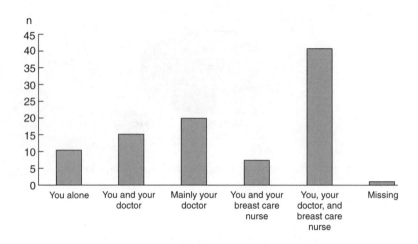

Fig. 5.9   Who do you feel made the treatment choice? Results of both the standard care and IVD groups combined.

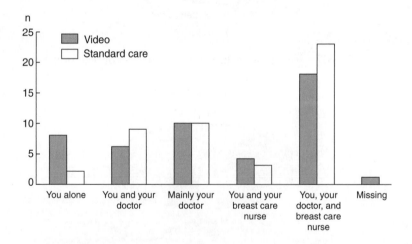

Fig. 5.10   Who do you feel made the treatment choice? Showing video vs standard care.

asked how they felt about the treatment decisions that were made overall, 75% were happy or very happy, with no statistical difference in either group. When asked their feelings about the amount of information they received overall, 72% of the patients were satisfied or very satisfied with the amount (Figs 5.11–5.12) and

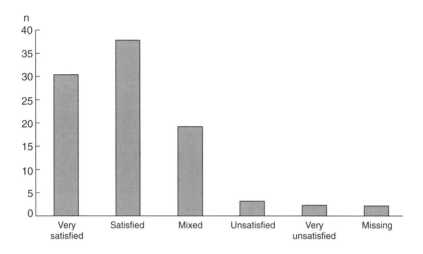

Fig. 5.11 Satisfaction with amount of information received—overall both IVD and standard care groups.

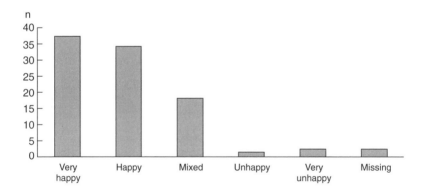

Fig. 5.12 Patients' feelings about the decision made—overall both IVD and standard care groups.

72% were satisfied or very satisfied with the quality of information received.

This study determined that providing information to women with early breast cancer using an interactive system did not significantly influence the anxiety and depression associated with its diagnosis and treatment in comparison with the best standard practice.

Both the control and experimental group demonstrated a significant reduction in anxiety by nine months post treatment. The study also determined that providing information using an IVD to women about treatment choices did not significantly increase their satisfaction with the choice they made. Both groups were largely satisfied with their choices and there was no statistically significant increase in the satisfaction expressed by the IVD group over the controls.

This study does demonstrate quite strongly the supportive role of the clinical nurse specialist (CNS) in breast care. Overall the patients in both groups of the study were satisfied with the tools used in information giving. Although the sources of information used varied in each arm of the study, the continuing support, both in terms of information and psychological support of the CNS, remained. Working together with the clinician it could be suggested that this support, rather than the tools used, was of primary importance. Luker *et al.* (1995) suggested detailed clinical information was not within the scope of the average ward nurse but may well fall within the scope of practice of the specialist breast care nurse. This study would appear to support that position. The fact that the CNS was seen by 50% of the patients as being involved in sharing in the decision-making process gives an indication of the strength of her input.

Overall, the IVD was evaluated very highly but it could be seen as being expensive in a number of ways. There is the initial capital purchase, the need for regular software updates, the need for a dedicated room during viewing of the program, and the associated manpower costs. The results of this study have indicated that viewing the IVD did not result in a significant increase in satisfaction or improvement in the intervention group's anxiety and depression scores over the group who received standard care, as both arms of the study were comparable.

It could be suggested that the comprehensive, individual support the patient received from the clinician, the CNS, and the multidisciplinary team was the key factor in satisfaction and adjustment, rather than the specific method of information-sharing used. If this is the case, and if cost is a major issue for carers provided the appropriate support from the clinician, CNS, and members of the multidisciplinary team is available to the patient, other less expensive forms of technical information support could be used to aid the provision of more detailed information. It could be suggested that literature, cards, other computer software, or a straight linear video dealing with specific scenarios could be just as effective as aids to information-giving.

The IVD has the ability to store and provide consistent protocol-based information at a uniformly high rate which would be difficult for a clinician or nurse to match, given the influence of the stresses of a working week. However, the professional has the ability to gauge a patients' mood and assess patient requirements which the machine cannot do (Maguire *et al.* 1980; 1983; Watson *et al.* 1988). It would be interesting to evaluate how the information given by the clinician and clinical nurse specialist varies as the week progresses and how other factors, e.g. time, stress, personal factors, affect the quantity and quality of information given to patients. This issue may be important when considering the debate on informed consent (Baum 1986; Baum and Houghton 1988; Williams 1992). With the IVD, professionals can demonstrate that a certain level of specific information was presented to the patient and that this was reinforced verbally by the CNS and in writing by the summary printout. The professional still has the problem of knowing exactly what impact stress and selective perception is having on the patient and therefore can never be sure exactly how much information the patient has absorbed. This, however, is balanced by the fact that in an imperfect world where no method of information-giving will be entirely correct for every patient, this system provides a useful vehicle for facilitating the informed consent process, not just for information in which risks and benefits must be assessed, but also for very technical information or in clinical trials (Williams 1992). The system could be useful to those conducting clinical trials by providing high-quality, evidence-based, personalized information which outlines the nature of clinical trials, the specifics of the trial, and the advantages the disadvantages of participation (Schafer 1989).

One important issue relates to the updating of software. Breast cancer research is constantly updating the information available and it will be important that any system or software has the capacity to incorporate new information at an affordable level. What is known and accepted today may need updating within a relatively short period. One solution could be an annual fee covering software updates which subscribers to the system could support. Although this study does not address the subject of the multitude of computer/CD systems available, it may be that in view of the fact that computer technology is advancing at such a rapid rate the principles used in the production and use of the IVD may be achieved more easily and less expensively today.

There is substantial research to support the view that good communication is important in patient adjustment to a cancer diagnosis (Maguire *et al.* 1978; 1980; 1982; 1983); the key players in the area of breast cancer appear to be the clinician (Maguire *et al.* 1978; Fallowfield *et al.* 1990*a,b*) and the breast care nurse (Maguire *et al.* 1980; 1982; 1983). It would appear that many patients do want access to good-quality information on their disease, treatment options, and side-effects (Thornton 1992; Maslin 1993; Maslin *et al.* 1993), and some patients, though not all, may wish to participate in the decision-making process (Bilodeau and Degner 1996). This study demonstrated that the IVD is highly evaluated by those who used it as a tool to assist decision-making. Those using the IVD system appeared very satisfied with the system, finding it easy to use. They did not appear to suffer any adverse psychological affects. Equally, this study showed that patients in the standard care group were very satisfied with their level of information. As suggested, this could mean providers of health care could opt for the simpler methods of reinforcing information-giving, provided the backbone of support and information is provided by healthcare professionals.

SDP/IVDs are not only about patient choice, they could also act as a valuable resource to standardize treatment protocols, promote evidence-based practice, and potentially help to collect valuable clinical and research data, and provide a measure for quality assurance (Kasper *et al.* 1992*a,b*; Mulley 1994; NHS Executive Clinical Outcomes Group for Breast Cancer Manual 1996; and Research Evidence 1996). It may be that these additional functions could provide a rationale for the expense incurred by the provision of these resources. The system could facilitate protocol-based practice but would this be acceptable to the majority of clinicians? It would be interesting to discover how many hospital-based consultants would support the introduction of such systems more widely. Can clinicians be induced to change their practice in line with the patient's expressed preference as result of using the

SDP? In this study with supportive clinicians the answer was 'yes', but this was equally true in the standard care group with the same consultants. Subjective experience seems to suggest that enthusiasts for SDP/IVDs are quality assurance officers, patient information groups, or nurses, the very people who may lack the authority or resources to make tangible changes in the health care system.

Is there then an added value in the use of IVD/SDPs in terms of data collection, quality assurance, and medical audit over time? This is a hypothesis that would need to be tested, but with compliance and cooperation in the use of the system it could be suggested that the system could provide a useful tool. It is possible that the IVD could act as a tool in helping to safeguard the multidisciplinary team from litigation because of its very specific and uniform delivery of information. As previously discussed, viewing the SDP ensures a quantifiable amount of information has been provided for the patient. It cannot ensure the information has been received but it can be used to substantiate the fact that certain information was covered. This could be useful, particularly in difficult situations such as patients giving consent to participate in clinical trials.

In summary, the IVD is an expensive tool in terms of capital cost, updates, and manpower in the provision of information to women with breast cancer. It would appear that the provision of psychological support and treatment information by a clinician and clinical nurse specialist trained in communication skills can provide an equally satisfactory service. It may be that if the IVD had been evaluated in a centre where the clinician was not open to dialogue with patients and where the services of a CNS was not available the results between the two groups could have been quite different.

The study also ascertained that the use of the IVD technology is acceptable to the women. The data from this study is helpful in that it demonstrated that the use of an IVD with explicit but empathetic information does not appear to be harmful to those women who choose to view it. For those patients who desire it, the IVD provides the opportunity to view personalized information which clearly outlines the risks and benefits of treatment options in an objective but empathetic manner, the content and quality of which is predetermined (Maslin *et al.* 1998 reproduced by kind permission of N.T. Research).

As noted earlier Maureen Roberts, Clinical Director of the Edinburgh Breast Screening project from 1979 to 1989, who succumbed to breast cancer, said

'Communication is all important. Proper truthful accounts of diagnosis, treatment and aftercare must be written and made available everywhere, so that women become well informed and most important, start to take part in the decision making process for themselves (Roberts 1998)'.

6

*Shared decision-making:
a summary and future issues*

A. Coulter

Time to act

Previous chapters in this book have argued the case for giving patients greater access to information and improving communication in clinical settings. There is also increasing enthusiasm for involving patients more closely in decisions about their care. The desire to encourage patient participation stems in part from a belief in the ethical principle of autonomy, but also from the hope that it will promote greater clinical effectiveness and more appropriate and efficient use of resources. It has long been known that there is a positive relationship between communication and clinical outcomes (Ley 1988; Simpson *et al.* 1991). There is also evidence that giving patients information and encouraging them to participate in treatment decisions can lead to improvements in doctor–patient relationships, health status, and quality of life (Brody *et al.* 1989; Lerman *et al.* 1990; Stewart 1995; Coulter 1997).

Yet many studies have shown that patients still find it difficult to obtain the information they need to participate in decisions about their care (Audit Commission 1993; Coulter *et al.* 1998). If the case for better information provision and a more participative style of decision-making is so overwhelming, why is it that clinical practice so often falls short of the ideal? What are the barriers to progress and how can they be overcome?

Three possible barriers are considered below—difficulties in knowing whether patients want to participate, uncertainties about the type of information patients need to help them determine their preferences, and problems with accessing suitable patient information materials to support decision-making. First though, it is important to be clear about the different approaches to clinical decision-making and the effects of changes in patients' expectations.

Models of decision-making

A hundred years ago doctors expected patients to follow their advice without question. Patients' views and preferences were seen as irrelevant and requests for additional information could be dismissed. In 1871 Oliver Wendell Holmes gave the following advice to American medical students (Laine and Davidoff 1996):

'Your patient has no more right to all the truth you know than he has to all the medicine in your saddlebags . . . He should get only just so much as is good for him . . .'.

Relationships between clinicians and patients are very different nowadays. Patients are more likely to challenge the notion that 'doctor knows best' and they expect to be given information about their condition and the treatment options. The doctor–patient relationship is undergoing a paradigm-shift away from the traditional paternalistic model towards a new form of decision-making which explicitly recognizes the patient's autonomy. The traditional model assumed that doctors and patients shared the same goals and that only the doctor was sufficiently informed and experienced to decide what should be done. Patient involvement was limited to giving or withholding consent to treatment.

A number of writers have described other models of decision-making which are now prevalent in clinical settings (Szasz and Hollender 1956; Veatch 1972; Quill 1983; Emanuel and Emanuel 1992; Deber 1994; Charles *et al.* 1997). At least four broad models of treatment decision-making can be distinguished: professional choice, consumer choice, the professional-as-agent, and shared decision-making (Table 6.1).

The consumer choice model is the polar opposite of the traditional or professional choice model, in that it assumes that the patient alone will make the decision once they have been provided with all necessary technical information. Thus the patient's preferences are pre-eminent and the clinician's role is reduced to that of providing technical information to support the patient's decision. The professional-as-agent model is somewhere between these two

Table 6.1 Models of clinical decision-making

Professional choice	Professional-as-agent	Shared decision-making	Consumer choice
Clinician decides, patient consents	Clinician elicits patient's views, then makes decision	Information shared, both decide together	Clinician informs, patient makes decision

extremes, in that it recognizes the importance of incorporating the patient's preferences into the process, but still leaves the clinician to make the final treatment decision. The clinician needs to ensure that the patient is informed about the options in order to elicit their preferences, but the decision remains with the clinician and is not, therefore, a shared one. In shared decision-making, however, the intention is that patients and health professionals share both the process of decision-making and ownership of the decision made. Shared information about values and likely treatment outcomes is an essential prerequisite, but the process also depends on a commitment from both parties to engage in the decision-making process. The clinician has to be prepared to acknowledge the legitimacy of the patient's preferences and the patient has to accept shared responsibility for the treatment decision.

It would be wrong to imply any value judgement about the relative desirability of the different models. All have their place in clinical situations—the trick is to match the appropriate decision-making style to the patient's needs at any particular time. For example, emergency situations often require clinicians to make quick decisions when there is no time to involve the patient. In these cases the professional choice model is entirely appropriate. In other situations it may be appropriate to leave the final decision to the patient, with the clinician's role relegated to provider of technical information as implied in the consumer choice model. Examples might include a woman's choice of contraceptive method: assuming she has full information about efficacy and risks and there are no relevant contra-indications, the patient who wants to should be allowed to decide for herself. In treating a condition like breast cancer, the clinician has to use his or her knowledge of the individual patient to determine the most appropriate style of decision-making. In most cases the choice will be between acting as the patient's agent by eliciting her preferences and using this information to decide on the most appropriate treatment, or adopting a shared decision-making style by actively involving her in the decision. The provision of reliable and clear information is central to both of these approaches.

Do patients want to participate in treatment decisions?

We know that patients want more information, but what is the evidence that they want to participate in decision-making? Failures in communication of information about illness and treatment are the most frequent source of patient dissatisfaction. There is plenty of evidence that patients want more information, but this does not necessarily mean that they want to participate in decision-making. A number of studies have investigated the extent of desire for participation among different groups of patients. For example, in a study of 439 interactions between adult cancer patients and oncologists in an American hospital, the majority (92%) preferred to be given all information including bad news, but only two-thirds (69%) said they wanted to participate in treatment decisions (Blanchard *et al.* 1988). A Canadian study looked at information and participation preferences among 52 outpatients undergoing post-surgical treatment for cancer (Sutherland *et al.* 1989). Almost two-thirds (63%) felt that the doctor should take the primary responsibility in decision-making, 27% felt it should be an equally shared process, and 10% felt they should take the major role.

Desire for participation has been found to vary according to age, educational status, disease group, and cultural background. A study of 256 American cancer patients found that younger patients were much more likely to want active participation in decisions about their care: 87% of patients aged under 40 expressed a desire to participate, compared with 62% of those aged 40–59 and 51% of those aged over 60 (Cassileth *et al.* 1980). The age differences in decision-making preferences suggest that the preference for active involvement may be increasing over time, reflecting greater knowledge of the risks as well as the benefits of medical care and decreased willingness to submit to the authority of clinicians.

Preference for an active role in decision-making may also vary according to the stage in the course of a disease episode and the severity of the patient's condition. Another Canadian study found a much greater desire for active participation among a randomly selected population sample than among a group of newly diagnosed cancer patients, pointing to the difficulty in predicting the level of involvement desired when serious illness strikes (Degner and Sloan 1992). There may also be important cultural differences. Studies comparing responses in different countries found that British breast cancer patients were less likely to prefer an active role than Canadian ones (Richards *et al.* 1995; Beaver *et al.* 1996). Although many patients want to participate in decision-making, it is important to remember that a substantial minority prefer a passive role.

What information do patients need to participate in decisions?

Many clinicians are attracted to the idea of a participative decision-making style in theory, but find it difficult to put into practice. Time constraints inhibit information provision and it is sometimes quite difficult to discover what the patient already knows and how much they want to be involved. Some clinicians fear that encouraging patients to choose between competing treatment options will place an additional burden on people who are feeling unwell and lead to unnecessary anxiety and distress. It is important to try to understand the patient's anxieties and to tailor communications accordingly.

Shared decision-making involves sharing information about the limitations and risks of treatment as well as the benefits. Patients with serious disease may prefer an optimistic rather than a realistic account of their chances of recovery. A Canadian study of patients with early-stage breast cancer found that patients' desire to adopt a positive approach to fighting their illness resulted in a tendency to want more aggressive interventions, notwithstanding the risks of the treatment (Charles *et al.* 1996). For example, patients tended to overestimate the possible benefits of chemotherapy and downplay the risks. If a more evidence-based approach to treatment decision-making is to be encouraged, it will be important to avoid the risk of undermining patients' coping strategies by invalidating their values and beliefs. Most of the cancer patients in the Canadian study preferred a shared decision-making style, but they were concerned about how blame for bad outcomes might be apportioned.

In cases of life-threatening illness it may be more important to allow patients an opportunity to express their concerns and preferences than to involve them in the decision itself. Studies in which breast cancer patients were offered a choice between mast-ectomy or breast-conserving surgery found no ill-effects of involving patients in the decision, but the findings conflicted on whether offering choice led to psychological benefits (Morris and Royle 1988; Wilson *et al.* 1988; Fallowfield *et al.* 1994*a*). Decision-making in cases of serious illness can be a protracted process. Patients require time to come to terms with the choices facing them and seek a sympathetic hearing from the clinician. Some-times consultation style may have a more important effect on the health outcome than the decision itself.

Patients require information for a variety of purposes. A quali-tative study of patients' information needs involving focus groups of patients with a variety of common conditions (not including breast cancer) identified a number of reasons why patients felt they needed information, including the following (Coulter *et al.* 1998):

- to explain what is wrong
- to get a realistic idea of prognosis
- to understand the processes and likely outcomes of tests and treatments
- to learn about available services
- to provide reassurance
- to help others (family, friends, carers, employers, etc.) understand
- to identify further information and sources of support.

Patients' information needs may change over the course of a disease. For example, at the time of first onset or diagnosis it may be more relevant to provide details of the tests and investiga-tions used and descriptive information about the condition and prognosis. Depending on the condition, it may be appropriate to provide detailed information about treatments at a later stage. A study designed to investigate the information needs of women newly diagnosed with breast cancer asked them to rank the relative importance of particular items of information (Luker *et al.* 1995). The items were ranked in the following order (most important first):

1. Information about the likelihood of cure from the disease.
2. Information about how advanced the disease is and how far it has spread.
3. Information about different types of treatment (surgical, chemotherapy, radiotherapy) and the advantages and disadvantages of each treatment.
4. Information about whether my children or other members of my family are at risk of getting breast cancer.
5. Information about unpleasant side-effects of treatment (for example, nausea, pain, change in physical appearance).
6. Information about how my family and close friends may be affected by the disease.
7. Information about caring for myself at home (for example, diet, support groups, help at home, social worker, counsellor).
8. Information about how the treatment may affect my ability to carry on my usual social activities (sports or hobbies, etc.).
9. Information about how the treatment may affect my feelings about my body and my sexual attractiveness (breast disfigurement, breast prosthesis, reconstructive surgery).

All these items of information are necessary if patients are to become active participants in decisions about their care. Some questions may be hard to answer because the information is uncertain or unavailable. An evidence-based approach is as important for patients as it is for clinicians, but this does not mean that lack of evidence justifies the omission of information about common treatments or possible outcomes. In the real world of clinical practice, decisions often have to be made on the basis of incomplete evidence and it is important that patients understand the inherent uncertainties.

How can patients' access to information be improved?

If decision-making is to be shared, the information to inform decisions must also be shared. Patients must be given help to obtain the information they need. Given the short consultation times experienced in most busy clinics, it is often unrealistic to expect clinicians to provide full information about the risks and benefits of all treatment options. This information is not always readily available to clinicians, let alone lay people. If patients are to be able to express their preferences, they require help in the form of user-friendly information packages and decision aids. Ideally this information should come from an independent source and be based on a sound overview of the scientific evidence. Such information is now available for certain diseases, but access to good quality patient information materials is still problematic.

Recent years have seen a rapid growth in the availability of patient information materials, including leaflets, videos, and multimedia technology, and of course the World Wide Web, which carries a huge amount of health information. We recently organized a study to assess the quality of patient information materials currently in use in the NHS. Fifty four materials giving information about common health problems, including leaflets, booklets, videos, and audiotapes, were reviewed by patient focus groups and by clinical specialists using structured checklists (Coulter *et al.* 1998). Publishers of the materials included consumer groups and voluntary organizations, drug companies, health authorities and NHS Trusts, commercial publishers, professional and academic bodies.

The results of the assessment were disturbing since they demonstrated that most of the materials fell far short of the standards required to support shared decision-making. Topics of relevance to patients were often omitted, technical terms were inadequately explained, coverage of treatment options was often incomplete, and many contained inaccurate and out-of-date information. They tended to provide a biased picture of treatment efficacy, providing much more information about benefits than risks and ignoring or glossing over uncertainties. Some materials were little more than advertising vehicles for a particular drug or organization and in many cases it was obvious that patients had not been consulted about their information needs prior to development of the materials.

The development of more sophisticated technologies for storing and accessing information will have a considerable impact on clinical practice in the future. Patients will become more knowledgeable and the availability of information will raise expectations. Currently only 7% of adults in Britain have access to the Internet, but this proportion is likely to grow fast. There are already more than 10 000 health-related web sites and more than a third of Internet users access the World Wide Web to retrieve health and medical information (Mitretek Systems 1997). Unfortunately the quality of information available from this source is no better, and sometimes much worse, than the materials reviewed in our study (Impicciatore *et al.* 1997). There is a risk that people will be seriously misinformed unless the quality improves. It will be important to develop some form of accreditation system to enable patients and clinicians to judge the reliability of health information.

Access to appropriate information can empower patients to express their treatment preferences and help professionals to improve the information base of clinical decisions, but if shared decision-making is to become a reality it will be necessary to develop the following resources:

(1) a supply of information materials for patients about treatment choices and outcomes based on scientifically valid, systematic reviews of the research evidence;

(2) a system for assessing the quality of the information materials before they are promulgated to patients;

(3) a means by which health authorities, provider units, clinicians, consumer health information services, and consumer groups can access the materials and make them available to patients;

(4) training programmes for clinicians and other information providers to help them elicit patients' preferences and use patient information materials effectively;

(5) a wide dissemination programme to tell patients about their rights to information and how to find it, and to encourage clinicians to provide it.

7

The breast care nurse

J. Secker Walker

The professional's dilemma

This section shares the personal views and experiences primarily of professionals when participating in the decision-making process. These accounts are complemented by short patient perspectives where possible. The views and perspectives they express are their own.

Facing choice

'A women must be offered every opportunity for full discussion and the involvement of a female counsellor who may help the woman understand and adjust to her diagnosis and treatments.'
(Kings Fund Consensus Statement 1986)

Recognition

The breast care nurse (BCN) usually meets the patient at the time of, or immediately after they have received, confirmation of the diagnosis of breast cancer. Before addressing the role played by the BCN in helping patients face the problems and dilemmas that accompany the diagnosis, it is important to recognize how they have reached the point of diagnosis and how each individual is responding to the impact of that diagnosis.

The woman may have been living with the unresolved, nagging suspicion that she could have breast cancer for several weeks or for only a few days. Patients awaiting investigation results are anxious and frightened and many describe this time of suspicion as the worst time of all (Maguire 1976).

In some 'one-stop' diagnostic clinics the results can be given the same day, but for most women the wait is usually more prolonged. The majority of women will have been told that 'one in ten' of all breast lumps is benign and that therefore the odds are in their favour; but however they rationalize, it is the possibility of being that 'one' that dominates their thinking. During this time some women are able to share their fears and mentally prepare. Other women remain isolated, shouldering the burden of worry alone, appearing to carry on as normal. The worry can provoke conflicting emotions:

- numbness
- disbelief
- protest
- anger
- despair
- fear
- hope.

In this turmoil, hope and fear see-saw; but fear is frequently uppermost. Fear for themselves, fear for their families, fear for the future. The more fatalistic expect that fate will throw them the loaded dice. This can also be true of many women with a family history: these women who have mentally prepared for an unfavourable result often express relief on hearing the confirming diagnosis. For most, however, hearing the actual diagnosis is a shock and is usually perceived as 'a catastrophic event tantamount to a death sentence' (Greer 1985).

The diagnosis

It is usually the responsibility of the specialist consultant to give the bad news. Giving the diagnosis of cancer is one of the most difficult duties of a doctor. However sensitively the diagnosis is presented, the stark words 'breast cancer' usually evoke emotion. Women respond to the news in different ways; they may be calmly accepting, blame themselves in some way, express anger, rage against fate, 'Why me?', or weep. It is known that patients retain very little of what is said at this time and that what they do retain can be extremely selective (Ley 1979). However, even those who in their stress cannot recall much detail after hearing the word 'cancer', later refer to the feel of the encounter. It matters to them whether the consultant looked them in the eye, whether their partner was included, and particularly whether or not they, the person, rather than the 'lump' were central to the discussion. The way the 'news' is given and how the doctor responds to the patient at this time can affect how the woman feels about and perceives her whole situation (Buckman 1992). It is important that the woman is reassured that although the diagnosis is a threat to life, death is not necessarily the end-point. She needs to be told that there are treatments and that there is hope. At diagnosis it is usually safe to express the hope of cure and that this is the aim of the surgical treatment of early breast cancer. Doctors have an undoubted duty at this time to state what they think would be the most appropriate treatment. It is important that the woman should feel valued as a person and to feel that the treatment chosen will be the best for her. Some doctors still presume to know what the patient wants and present treatment and make decisions without meaningful consultation (Morris 1983).

Jane: 'One of the worst things about having cancer was the feeling that I no longer owned my body; worse still was the feeling that my mind was also superfluous'.

However, some women bow under the weight of the diagnosis and completely abdicate responsibility for their treatment. Others expect, and many need, to have their wishes considered. Where there is treatment choice, the doctor should explain the options and allow the woman the opportunity to participate in the decision-making process (Degner and Sloan 1992; Alderson *et al.* 1994). The diagnosis of cancer takes away the feeling of personal control that everyone needs to get on with their daily lives. Some women are intensely aware of this feeling. They recognize their need and are increasingly demanding to share in the decision-making process as one way of regaining a measure of that control. The decision they are about to make can have a profound effect on their life. They usually need more information and further time to consider all the implications of each choice. The person who can provide both the time and the relevant information is the breast care nurse (Cotton *et al.* 1991).

The Role of the breast care nurse (BCN)
The BCN has specialist training (Maguire *et al.* 1980; 1982; 1983; Maguire and Faulkner 1988*a*,*b*,*c*; Maguire 1990; Watson *et al.* 1988)

to help the patient at this time and throughout her treatment. She is an integral part of the breast care team and her role is to provide adequate psychological assessment of individual need, appropriate information, practical help, emotional support, and, when necessary, to act as an advocate on behalf of the patient (Cancer Relief Macmillan Fund 1994). When the BCN first meets a women newly diagnosed with breast cancer she is often faced with a person at a crisis point in their life. A person in 'crisis' as someone exhibiting the following characteristics:

- emotional shock
- a need to change one's behaviour
- a need for immediate action or intervention
- the confrontation of a totally new phenomenon
- the loss of the ability to think rationally or to integrate new information
- a breakdown in the person's system of values
- a feeling of having reached a 'dead end' with no sense of how to proceed
- unpredictability—both for the person who experiences the crisis and those who observe the situation (Kfir 1989).

Many, if not all, of these characteristics are exhibited by breast cancer patients at diagnosis.

Support

> 'Give sorrow words: the grief that does not speak
> Whispers the o'er fraught heart, and bids it break.'
> (William Shakespeare, *Macbeth*)

At this time of 'crisis' for the patient, the BCN needs to be particularly sensitive to her personal priorities. The woman may feel overwhelmed by the news. A quiet place should be provided where she and any companions can be private. Many women appreciate being given the opportunity to be alone for a while, to collect thoughts or vent feelings without the presence of a stranger. Others are grateful for the presence of the nurse.

'Tea and Sympathy' is not out of place; many women are shocked and numbed and they need nurturing. The patient may need to be encouraged to express her feelings; she may wish to retell her story, share her pain, or simply require a shoulder to cry on. The nurse should convey a friendly interest in the woman as a person and respond to her with empathy. This is probably not an appropriate time to either formally 'counsel' or to diligently inform; often all that is required is support. The BCN should present herself as someone who will be available to continue to support the patient throughout her treatment, and as someone with specialist knowledge who may be able to help the patient have a clearer understanding of her disease and its treatment. The intervention of a specially trained breast care nurse can improve a patient's knowledge and decrease her level of anxiety (Wilkinson *et al.* 1988).

In her book, *Coping with breast cancer*, Heyderman (1996) writes of her personal experience as a breast cancer patient and of meeting the BCN.

'People assume that if you are a doctor, you know all the answers and don't need reassurance. I had lots of questions but I knew first hand just how busy and overworked my doctors were ... I felt I could let my hair down in front of another woman, cry and say things I had been bottling up, not wanting to bother my doctors or worry my family ... I was as worried and distressed as any other woman with breast cancer.'

Some patients may be too distressed to take in further information and need time to assimilate the news. It may be appropriate to give written information to take home, a telephone contact number, and possibly make an appointment for another day when these topics could be discussed and the patient's questions answered. There are some patients who need to know, there and then, what the future might hold. It is therefore important for the BCN to assess the impact of the diagnosis for that individual patient and how she appears to be coping psychologically.

Assessment

How is this woman coping? When people are under stress, 'a state when the demands on a person exceed his or her capacity to respond (Rowland 1989)', there are various ways in which they

y react. Greer and Watson (1987) have identified different
ping styles:

'helpless/hopeless'—these patients tend to 'give up' in the face of
cancer. They feel overwhelmed by the disease and make little
effort to cope or adjust.

'fatalism'—these patients acknowledge the seriousness of their
disease but accept it as their lot, with little or no show of emotional
distress, and carry on with their lives much as before.

'positive avoidance'—these patients 'play down' the threat of the
disease. Though aware of the nature of the disease, they avoid
dwelling on the subject. They too want to carry on as normal.

'fighting spirit'—these patients rise to the challenge of overcoming
cancer.

'anxious preoccupation'—these patients are often in such a state
of heightened awareness about the disease that they are unable to
think objectively.

   Many patients are ambivalent about how they 'really' feel and
may experience more than one coping style, as they are not
mutually exclusive. Experience has shown that it is usually
women who display 'fighting spirit' or who are overtly pre-
occupied by the disease who are most anxious to be involved in
the decision-making process. They find out as much as possible
and are aware of how the disease may impact on their lives. They
recognize that, in all probability, life will always be defined by
this diagnosis and can have far-reaching consequences.

Linda: 'From here on I knew my life would never be the same,
         even if I survived what was about to go through phys-
         ically, mentally and emotionally would mean I could
         never be the same person . . . and I loved who I was.
         I knew myself very well, what I could cope with, my
         weaknesses and my strengths. I was enjoying life, every
         aspect of my life was complete and happy. I had worked
         hard to get to that point in my life. Now I was being
         forced into unknown territory and I didn't want to go . . .
         but I didn't want to die and that's the bottom line.'

Linda writes of being forced into 'unknown territory.' Her whole person is threatened.

Breast cancer diagnosis may be seen by patients to:

- threaten their life
- threaten their femininity
- threaten their family
- produce a fear of being stigmatized or even rejected once the diagnosis is known.

There is the immediate worry: 'has the cancer spread?'. There is the ongoing uncertainty over the future and how this uncertainty could impact on relationships, children, employment, and many other aspects of the patient's life. There is the possibility that treatment could seriously affect the ability of the woman to continue with her normal daily activities (Holland and Rowland 1989). All these threats are going to impact on a whole range of issues, including what to do about treatment.

Facilitating surgical choice

'Patients, families and carers should be given clear information and assistance in a form they can understand about treatment options and outcomes available to them from diagnosis onwards.'

(The Calman Report 1995)

Information

Many women feel rushed into a decision regarding treatment without being sufficiently well informed. Doctors frequently underestimate the amount of information their patients want and most women want more than many doctors provide (Waitzkin 1984). They require more information before either agreeing to a proposed treatment plan or participating in choice (Royal College of Nursing 1994). The information should be provided in a simple, staged way and in a form and manner which helps the patient understand the disease, the rationale of the surgical treatment choice, and the psychological impact of all treatment of breast cancer (Fallowfield *et al.* 1990a; Department of Health 1990).

Such information can help women to re-appraise the nature of the disease and possibly to face the future with more optimism.

Carol: 'I was given a lot of information about my different treatment options and came home armed with masses of leaflets, which I found hard to take in at first, but I was grateful that I had been given the opportunity to discuss the options with the counsellor . . . and the opportunity of making an informed decision that was going to have a tremendous impact on my body and my life.'

If the woman is comfortable with the surgical choice proposed by the doctor, the BCN should make sure that:

(1) the patient has considered the possible surgical options;
(2) the surgery proposed is truly what the patient wants;
(3) the patient understands what it entails and is aware of any possible side-effects.

Choices

Surgery is the orthodox treatment for women presenting with early breast cancer. The aim is to achieve local control of the disease and cure where possible. The surgical choices are:

- local excision ('lumpectomy') and radiotherapy
- mastectomy
- mastectomy and reconstruction
- axillary dissection?
- no surgery!

It is important to remember and acknowledge that most woman who develop breast cancer are usually otherwise fit and well and that the treatments offered are going to change that state. They will become 'unwell' for varying lengths of time and by varying degrees. A serious consideration for some women will be how the various treatments are going to impact on their lives. The most appropriate treatment will depend on many factors including the patient's circumstances, personality, expectations, fears, beliefs, values, and cultural background.

Doctor: 'If you were my wife, this is what I would advise.'

A proposed treatment can sometimes be presented to a patient in this format. This may seem coercive but some women welcome such directional advice and is why they have sought a specialist opinion; indeed the very intimacy of the statement can make them feel valued. Others might feel it was patronizing. A wise doctor will assess whether a woman wants to be dealt with honestly and openly as an equal or prefer to be directed more strongly. At the end of the second millennium, it might be safer assume that a woman expects to be treated as an equal in decision-making unless she positively states otherwise! However, as discussed earlier, some research has shown that what patients want most is information and discussion of the treatments rather than necessarily wanting to make the ultimate treatment decision (Degner and Sloane 1992; Hack *et al.* 1994; Richards *et al.* 1995).

Carol: 'It was very important to me to feel that I had choices after being diagnosed with breast cancer, and to have an element of control over what was happening to me. It was essential that I didn't feel a helpless victim.'

1. 'Lumpectomy'

For many women there is no contest; for them conserving surgery was always their first choice and if it is appropriate in their case they feel fortunate. These women are often highly concerned about their physical appearance and maintaining their body image (Ashcroft *et al.* 1985). In most cases, breast conserving surgery leaves the woman with only a faint scar on a breast which is usually cosmetically acceptable. It is important for women to appreciate that conserving the breast can only safely be offered with the addition of postoperative radiotherapy, and that radiotherapy itself is not without side-effects that could affect body image. This is an area that often requires clarification and where the BCN can provide information regarding possible side-effects, what the therapy actually involves, the timing of the therapy after surgery, the number of weeks taken, and the frequency of the treatments. The whole scenario is often a surprise to patients but many consider that this option is preferable to a mastectomy, even if attending for the therapy involves a long journey with possible disruption to family, work, and social activities.

Maja: 'When you are told you have breast cancer, you'll do anything to preserve your life and if that means a mastectomy, yes, you'll do it. But when you have the time to consider and realize that you can conserve the breast and have an equal chance of survival, then other considerations come into play: how you feel about that breast and the risk of the cancer coming back in that breast.'

2. Mastectomy

About 30% of women offered choice opt for a mastectomy (Fallowfield *et al.* 1990*a*). However, before doing so they should receive sufficient counselling concerning both the physical and psychological impact of the surgery (Maguire *et al.* 1980). Implicit in the choice is an acceptance of a serious change in body image (Wilson *et al.* 1988), but many are unprepared for the lack of, or altered, skin sensation. All will experience a time of 'mourning' before they can fully come to terms with the loss.

Choosing mastectomy

Carol: 'I was given a choice of a mastectomy, with immediate reconstruction if I wished, or just have the lump removed, followed by radiotherapy. Either way I was to have the lymph nodes removed as well. My first reaction was to keep the breast at all costs. I had always lacked confidence about my appearance because I have spina bifida and scoliosis. To lose a breast as well seemed too awful to contemplate. I considered my breasts to be the best part of my body. I came home with my husband in a daze, armed with various booklets which I read over the next few days . . . while in a state of shock I was going to have to make the most important decision of my life. The more I read the more I came round to thinking that the mastectomy was the right choice for me. I made a list of 'for' and 'against'. The 'for' column was extremely practical; the 'against' was purely emotional. My practical side won. I based my decision on two things: if I just had the lump removed I would constantly have worried about cancer returning in the same breast, and secondly because of my disability my energy levels are very low, and I didn't feel that physically I could cope with radiotherapy, which would have to be done on a daily basis for six weeks, involving a long car journey to the hospital. So the decision was made, and my husband whole-heartedly supported me.'

Carol had always been a battler; she had always worked, was married, and had a child. She is determined to continue to lead a full and active life—and to do that she needed to have a measure of control over what happened to her. Carol elected to have reconstruction. Women can have many different and valid reasons for choosing not to have breast-conserving surgery:

- fear of recurrence
- fear of radiotherapy
- fear of cosmetic distortion
- shortest treatment time
- personal belief.

1. The predominant reason is fear of recurrence. Some women feel safer when the whole breast is removed and therefore the known risk of local recurrence greatly reduced. They do not want to be constantly worrying 'is there anything there?' A frequent reaction at diagnosis is to want to get rid of the part that has 'gone rotten', that has let them down in some way.

2. Some women have a horror of radiotherapy and what it involves. This may be from reading, hearsay, or a recalled childhood experience. Others confuse radiotherapy and chemotherapy. Explanation and counselling may help to allay many of the fears and misconceptions but for some, if the necessity for radiotherapy is greatly reduced by mastectomy, then that is the option of choice.

3. Fear of cosmetic distortion can be a serious consideration for those women for whom a 'lumpectomy' may not conserve enough of the breast, i.e. the removal of a relatively large lump from a small breast or a quadrant from a large breast. Mastectomy or mastectomy plus reconstruction is often a preferred choice.

4. Possibly the shortest treatment time is mastectomy, where the need for radiotherapy is greatly reduced. This can be valid for

women who have a chronic dislike of hospitals, who may feel too old to 'be fussed' by prolonged treatment, or who may feel that the shortest treatment route will allow them to 'get on with their lives' more quickly.

5. Personal knowledge of a breast cancer patient who survived following mastectomy can be a powerful reason for some women to follow the same course of action. If this belief is compounded by knowledge of another woman who had the alternative treatment and who subsequently died, then the woman is often adamant that mastectomy must be the 'right' treatment.

Choosing not to have reconstruction For clinical reasons some women are advised against reconstruction. Others who have the choice, refuse. Women can have physical, psychological, emotional, or social reasons for choosing not to have reconstruction:

- some find the thought of an implant repugnant
- some are influenced by adverse press reports of implants
- some feel there is less to go wrong
- some women who are old or who are not sexually active may feel that it is not necessary
- some prefer to live with the mastectomy scar and see how they feel about it, and maybe reconsider later
- some do express a need for time to 'mourn' the loss of the breast, the loss being seen as an outward sign of an inner grief
- some need to 'front' what cancer has done to them and if that means a mastectomy, then so be it; these women also often choose not to wear an external prosthesis for much the same reason
- some find length of time to complete the reconstruction unacceptable.

3. Mastectomy and reconstruction
'We restore, repair and make whole those parts which nature has given and fortune taken away. Not so much that they may delight the eye but that they may buoy the spirit and help the mind of the afflicted.'

(Gasper Tagliacozzi 1597)

The ability of surgeons to offer immediate or delayed reconstruction of the breast makes the mastectomy option more attractive for many women. Where mastectomy isn't an option but a surgical necessity, it can possibly make the contemplation of the 'loss' less traumatic. Research has shown (Dean *et al.* 1983) that problems associated with denial, anger, and sorrow at the loss of a breast are alleviated by reconstruction and that these women have significantly less psychological morbidity. Breast reconstruction, however skilled, cannot replicate the feel and texture of the 'real thing'. It is important for women to understand this: many get carried along by the surgeon's enthusiasm for their art and can be disappointed when the reality does not match their personal expectation.

When counselling women who are contemplating any form of reconstruction, it is wise to begin by helping the patient understand mastectomy, to look at photographs and then help her to the realization that reconstruction is an imperfect alternative to a flat chest, rather than a perfect replacement. Understandably many women (and their partners too) confuse breast reconstruction with breast enhancement. It can be another blow to their diminishing self-esteem when they are shown the reality. Medical photographs are by definition not 'glamour shots', but explained with sensitivity can help in the realistic preparation for surgery. It is sometimes useful for potential patients to speak to or meet women who have had reconstruction. This should be tempered with caution; first, because often it is only those women who are extremely pleased with the result who volunteer and secondly, it has been known for women to use the occasion to inappropriately 'off-load' other possibly unrelated problems. The woman making the choice needs to have a balanced view of the advantages and disadvantages of reconstruction and the different sorts available. It is essential for the BCN to assess the underlying emotional and physical reasons for each woman wishing to undergo breast reconstruction. It is preferable that the decision to go ahead with reconstruction should be the result of consideration of her own personal need and not at the behest of, or to please, her partner or another person.

Women have many dilemmas when contemplating this form of surgery. Immediate or delayed reconstruction may depend on the availability of surgeons. Some women fear that they may be putting themselves at risk by a reconstruction that involves an implant: an alternative method which may involve transfer of tissue and the skill of a specialist plastic surgeon could mean a time delay of many months or sometimes years. This may be acceptable to some but not to others for whom immediacy is a prime concern. Time must be taken by both the surgeon and the nurse to explain the choices carefully, to discover the areas of concern, and to clarify where there is confusion or possibly misinformation, thus enabling the woman to be comfortable with her final decision.

4. Axillary dissection

As women become better informed about breast cancer and its treatment, they learn that breast cancer is more than one disease and that not all cancers necessarily require all the standard treatments. Dissection of the axilla with the attendant problem of the possibility of lymphoedema is an area of clinical uncertainty and patient concern. Traditionally, the axilla was dissected in order to gain the greatest amount of prognostic information. The dissection allowed the histopathologist to report on the condition and involvement of the axillary nodes. Surgeons are now exploring other methods of obtaining the same information. Radiographic identification of the sentinel node and the use of MRI are two methods currently being researched. To date, nothing is as definitive as surgery and most women accept the need and recognize the risk; for others, the risk of developing lymphoedema would so impinge on their quality of life, that having weighed the benefits and the risks, they accept responsibility for their part in the surgical decision.

5. No treatment

Rosie: 'My body is my temple.'

Rosie was an extremely angry yoga teacher who felt that the diagnosis of breast cancer was a personal affront to both her and her lifestyle. She contacted her eminent guru in India, who advised 'your mind is strong, you know your body, you know what to eat, continue living as usual and take everything that western medicine can offer'. This is a useful story to relate when confronted by a woman who may be considering rejecting conventional medicine. It is difficult not to be coercive after seeing the distressing consequences of refusing conventional treatment for primary breast cancer. These women frequently talk of the need for a holistic approach to their treatment, feeling that this will only be offered outside conventional medicine. Sometimes all that is required for them to accept primary treatment is a little reassurance that many therapies that were previously considered to be in the 'alternative' domain are now being used as part of complementary cancer care. The emphasis being complementary; meaning in addition to, not an alternative to, conventional medicine.

Occasionally women balk at the thought of any form of interventionist medical treatment and opt to explore 'alternative' methods. It is ethically proper to advise these women that the 'no treatment' choice is the only one that offers no hope of 'cure' and that this is not an option considered by health professionals working in mainstream evidence-based medicine. By delaying or rejecting conventional treatment women are putting themselves at greater risk, and their decision may also cause additional distress to their family, carers, and friends. However, should these women chose to seek alternative medicine, it is beholden on the health professionals to assure them that the decision does in no way prejudice them from seeking conventional treatment at a subsequent time.

Adjuvant systemic therapy

Adjuvant therapy is still evolving and the treatment recommended consequently changes with scientific review, but nearly all women with high or moderate risk of recurrence will be offered some form of systemic treatment. Generally all postmenopausal women are offered hormonal treatment and for those with high nodal involvement and an aggressive tumour, chemotherapy may also be considered. The recent overview shows that premenopausal women with hormone-sensitive tumours can equally benefit from hormone therapy (Early Breast Cancer Trialists' Collaborative Group (EBCTCG) 1998). Chemotherapy is usually offered to premenopausal women with any adverse histology (EBCTCG 1992).

After the maelstrom of emotions that women experience at diagnosis and during the early days prior to surgery, the time following surgery can be one of calm reassessment for some women. Others experience enormous relief, even euphoria. They have survived the first hurdle. However, these see-saw emotions, fear and hope, are again felt by many awaiting the histology results. These results are seen as the key of future treatment and a 'clue' to prognosis.

Carol: 'On the day I was discharged I had the wonderful news that all 11 lymph nodes were clear. The relief was enormous. It was debated as to whether I should have chemotherapy as an additional backup and the decision was left to me. I decided to have it. I wanted to give myself the best chance possible.'

This is the 'bottom line' for many women; if there is just the remotest chance that they may benefit from adjuvant therapy, they will take it (Slevin *et al.* 1990). And there's the rub; it is unknown who will and who will not benefit from adjuvant therapy. It is this uncertainty that makes informed 'choice' extremely difficult. The need for some form of systemic treatment has to be handled sensitively. The very idea that there could still be malignant cells at large which have the potential to threaten life is intellectually and emotionally too difficult for some women. However, if a relationship of trust and openness has been established between the patient and the BCN, the complex issue of the possibility of micrometastases can usually be discussed.

Chemotherapy

'Life is just one damned thing after another.'
(Elbert Hubbard 1859–1915)

For many women, having to face the possibility that they may benefit from chemotherapy finally brings home the seriousness of their condition. As one previously phlegmatic women remarked, 'this is really grown-up time!'. The BCN should help the women to explore their fears, both concerning the treatment and its meaning for them individually. When a women is considering chemotherapy she has to weigh the possible long-term benefit against the known, mostly short-term, adverse side-effects. On the whole, patients tend to overestimate the magnitude of treatment benefit and underestimate the toxicity of chemotherapy (Siminoff *et al.* 1989). The BCN can assist the woman to have a more realistic approach, although many women are never at ease with the concept that they will never know whether the treatment they choose will benefit them personally or whether they didn't need it in the first place, as they may already be 'cured' by the surgical intervention. The side-effects of chemotherapy vary in intensity with different regimes, and individual women react differently. The toxicity and the consequent side-effects are accepted as a necessary evil by women who feel they must 'go for broke'. The knowledge that most side-effects are temporary and reversible are deciding factors for a lot of women. However, many side-effects can seriously disturb the quality of life for these women, affecting their well-being, their body image, and their ability to get on with daily living. The most common side-effects are nausea, loss of appetite, mouth soreness, hair loss, and problems associated with a low blood count. These problems include fatigue, being prone to bruising or bleeding, and being more susceptible to infection. In some premenopausal women, chemotherapy may trigger an early menopause; in others, ovulation may cease permanently with resultant infertility. This is particularly the case for women over 40 years old.

'Speak to us of children ... They are the sons and daughters of life's longing for itself.'

(Kahil Gibran 1926)

The risk of permanent damage to the ovaries depends on age and the drugs used, as well as the timing and duration of the therapy. Fertility is more likely to return to normal in younger woman. It may take as long as two years after treatment for normal periods to return (EBCTCG 1992), although resuming menstruation does not always mean a woman is ovulating. The possible risk of infertility can be an enormous issue for many young women who may wish to contemplate a family or increase an existing one. This is an area that needs skilled counselling prior to deciding on which treatment regime and what level of toxicity. When presented with a treatment option that is aimed at saving her life, the woman may feel beholden to comply with whatever is suggested, or may feel too intimidated to disclose her particular concerns to the doctor. Oncologists are usually sensitive to the woman's needs but this may not always be so and occasionally the BCN may need to intercede and bring these concerns to the doctor's attention.

Adjuvant hormonal therapy

The efficacy of hormonal manipulation in the treatment of breast cancer is well established. A major advance in the management of breast cancer has been the use of the drug tamoxifen.

Tamoxifen

Tamoxifen has been given as a treatment for breast cancer since 1973. It was initially prescribed for patients with advanced disease and it has been taken by over four million women. It is a hormone that works as an oestrogen antagonist and blocks the receptor sites on breast cancer cells, but the effect seems to be confined to those cells; elsewhere in the body it appears to act as a mild oestrogen. Many clinical trials and much research has been undertaken to determine the risk to the human body, and the dose of 20 mg/day has been shown to reduce the risk of local recurrence, reduce the risk of developing cancer in the contralateral breast, and to significantly improve survival by up to 25% (EBCTCG 1992). It is essential that the BCN gives careful explanation, counselling, and appropriate information leaflets to those women for whom tamoxifen is the considered medical adjuvant treatment choice. Most women agree to the treatment, while some need time to consider, and others refuse.

Choosing not to take tamoxifen

Women choose not to take tamoxifen usually because they consider the possible side-effects unacceptable. Many have been influenced by adverse media coverage of the drug. The latest published research (EBCTCG 1998) has been reported more positively, and women appear to be responding similarly. However, for some women taking a drug daily for the recommended five years is unacceptable. Compared to chemotherapy, hormonal treatment is far less toxic, the side-effects are fairly mild, are usually few, and tend to subside with time. The most common side-effects are slight indigestion or nausea, dizziness, weight gain, and menopausal symptoms such as hot flushes and sweats, vaginal dryness, and mood changes. The adverse side-effect highlighted by the media was the increase in endometrial cancer in postmenopausal women. Naturally women were alarmed. For them it did not make sense to treat one cancer by putting them at risk of developing another. Even after careful counselling that tamoxifen prevents 30 times more cancer than it causes and an appreciation of the absolute risk, the cost-benefit trade off is still unacceptable to some women. Some women begin chemotherapy and taking tamoxifen at the same time; others not until the completion of chemotherapy. These women will have been having some form of active treatment for nine months or more and feel that enough has already been done to combat the disease. It is now time to get on with life. Further medication would be a constant reminder they would rather forego.

Choosing to discontinue tamoxifen

Many patients have problems with sexuality, both during and after treatment. They have breast cancer and their recent life has been defined by that disease and its treatment. They may feel a loss of femininity and that their role as a wife/partner has changed. Adverse effects of tamoxifen can be the 'last straw'. These patients need to be given the opportunity to discuss their feelings. The BCN can support, reassure, counsel, advise, and where appropriate suggest the help of relevant outside agencies. Women who feel that taking tamoxifen is seriously interfering with their quality of life should be encouraged to discuss the problem with a specialist doctor. The doctor and patient can together decide how best to proceed.

Clinical trials

'When a lot of remedies are suggested for a disease, that means it can't be cured.'

(Anton Chekhov, *The Cherry Orchard*)

Major advances have been made to improve the outcome for women with breast cancer. This has been possible only after each advance has been demonstrated to be of clear value in carefully conducted clinical trials. Women with breast cancer who are asked to participate in clinical trials need to be accurately informed by the clinician. It is the duty of the doctor to explain the nature of the trial, what randomization means, the possible treatment scenarios, and their implication for the patient. It is very hard for women who have struggled to accept the need for adjuvant therapy to then be asked to take what can appear to be 'pot-luck' in a clinical trial. It is imperative that they understand that their treatment is not compromised. Sharing in treatment decision-making frequently involves considering clinical trials. The patients are being asked to make difficult choices at a time when they are physically and emotionally vulnerable. The BCN can support the patient and encourage her to express any doubts and confusions. The nurse can often present the complexities of a trial in a manner that the patient may find easier to understand and often can give the patient more time to consider all the options and their implications. She can inform and support the patient; however, it is not her role to advise or in any way coerce. Whether or not to enter a clinical trial is the patient's choice alone. The nurse should support the patient in her decision and through any subsequent treatment (Royal College of Nursing 1988).

Conclusion

'If the women is fully informed in decisions about her own care without feeling patronised she is more likely to feel positive about the treatment she elects, however distasteful it might be.'

(Kings Fund Consensus Statement 1986)

The BCN works most successfully when a relationship of mutual trust and respect exists between the nurse and clinician. The patient can then feel secure in the knowledge that the BCN is an essential member of a team which is working together to help her. Patients are being asked to make difficult choices at a time when they are physically and emotionally vulnerable. The intervention of specially trained nurses can improve patients' knowledge and decrease their level of anxiety. This is essential if the patient is to successfully participate in the decision-making process. Participating in the process does not necessarily guarantee contentment with choice. Where a choice is subsequently unsuccessful, it can induce feelings of blame and regret. With the knowledge of hindsight, other patients may regret their decision. However, most patients are satisfied that they made an informed decision.

Maja: 'I made the right choice for me and I don't ever regret it.'

8

Decision-making in breast cancer screening

R. Given-Wilson

Breast cancer screening can involve difficult choices, both for women being screened and for doctors working in screening. I will discuss the current evidence about the value of screening, how it works, what women and doctors can expect from the screening process, and the decisions that must be made.

Why screen for breast cancer?

The purpose of screening is to reduce the mortality from breast cancer. The value of regular screening for women over 50 years old has been demonstrated by rigorous randomized controlled trials. To examine this evidence in more detail we need first to look at the breast cancer situation current in the UK. Breast cancer is the commonest cancer in women in this country and it is estimated one in 12 women will develop breast cancer during their lives. In 1991 34 500 women were newly diagnosed with breast cancer in the UK. 80% of cases occur in postmenopausal women (Cancer Research Campaign 1996).

There are a number of risk factors related to breast cancer (Table 8.1), the strongest risk factors are being female and an older age. Most of the well-established risk factors for breast cancer are not modifiable. Unlike the association between smoking and lung cancer there is no single major cause of breast cancer that can be easily avoided.

Treatment for breast cancer, both local and systemic, shows success rates closely linked to the stage of the cancer at presentation (Fig. 8.1) (Cancer Research Campaign 1996). Patients with small tumours which are less than 2 cm in diameter have a greater

Table 8.1 Factors associated with an increased risk of developing breast cancer

---

- Female sex
- Increasing age
- Family history
- Previous history of breast cancer
- Certain types of benign dysplasias proved on biopsy (e.g. atypical ductal hyperplasia, multiple papillomatosis)
- Reproductive factors: early age of menarche, nulliparity, late age at first birth (>30 years), late age at menopause
- Rare, inherited familial syndromes (e.g. Li Fraumeni syndrome)
- Ionizing radiation

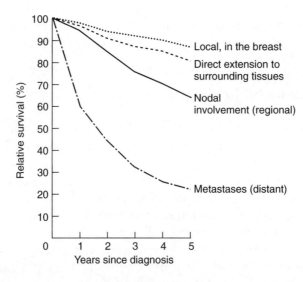

Fig. 8.1 Five-year relative survival for patients aged 15–74 years diagnosed in south east England 1986–9.

than 90% chance of surviving 5 years, compared with 60% for patients with tumours over 5 cm in diameter. Involvement of axillary nodes indicates a worse progress (Miller *et al.* 1995). It therefore seems logical to think of early detection by screening as a way of reducing breast cancer deaths. The rational for this is that, as survival after treatment and diagnosis is directly related to stage of diagnosis, so the earlier that the breast cancer can be diagnosed, the better the survival rate.

There are a number of biases which may affect the evaluation of a screening programme. These can be overcome by using careful randomized controlled trials to assess the value of mammographic breast screening. Such trials compare the relative risk of dying from breast cancer in women invited for screening over a number of years with the risk in a similar group of women not invited for screening. For women aged 50 years and over at entry, all trials show a reduction in cancer mortality by 20–39%, although the results are not statistically significant in all cases (Fig. 8.2). For women aged 40–49 years, evidence for the benefit of screening is less convincing. Trials do not show a statistically significant reduction in breast cancer mortality in these women after seven to ten years of follow-up but after ten years of follow-up there is a non-significant trend toward a reduced mortality of between 13 and 23% in several studies (Wald *et al.* 1993). This has led to controversy about the benefit of screening mammography in women aged 40–49. Several meta-analyses of screening women under the age of 50 have provided conflicting evidence about mortality reduction. Part of the difficulty in evaluating

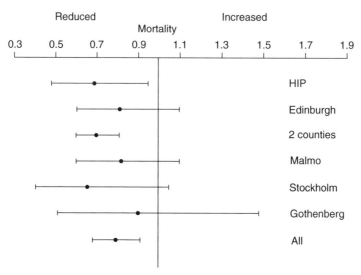

Fig. 8.2 Relative risk of mortality from breast cancer in women aged 50–74 invited for screening (RCT).

screening among younger women is that the number of women aged 49 and under included in large studies has been too small to allow proper subgroup analysis of the effect of screening and a definitive trial is awaited.

How the National Health Service Breast Screening Programme (NHSBSP) began

In 1986 a working group chaired by Professor Sir Patrick Forrest published a report on breast cancer screening (Forrest 1986). It had examined the evidence from two published randomized controlled trials, the initial data from the UK randomized controlled trials, and data from other non-randomized studies. It concluded that deaths from breast cancer in women aged 50–64 years who are offered screening by mammography could be reduced by one-third or more. The group recommended the setting up by the NHS of a nationwide programme of mammographic screening (Table 8.2). The Forrest Committee's recommendations were accepted and the National Health Service Breast Screening Programme (NHSBSP) began screening in 1988. In 1995 two view mammography was adopted for prevalent screens after a randomized controlled trial run under the auspices of the UKCCCR (United Kingdom Coordinating Committee on Cancer Research) showed 24% higher cancer detection rates with two views (Wald *et al.* 1995). Apart from this change, the programme still follows the guidelines laid down by Forrest, although the age

Table 8.2 Recommendations of the Forrest Committee on breast cancer screening (Forrest 1986) and current NHSBSP guidelines

- Target population: women aged 50–64 years by direct invitation, women aged 65 and over may be screened on request. (The NHSBSP has agreed to increase the upper age limit to 69 for invited women and is running demonstration projects to assess the impact of doing so. There is a multicentre trial screening women aged 40–49 taking place under the auspices of the NHSBSP.)
- Interval: three years (evaluation of annual vs three-yearly mammography is ongoing)
- Number of views: single mediolateral oblique view. (Since 1995, two-view mammography has been instituted for the prevalent (first) screen. Single-view continues to be undertaken for incident (subsequent) screens, but remains under review.)

limits for screening and the frequency of screening as well as the number of views for incident screens are all being studied within the auspices of the programme and may be changed.

How is screening organized?

Within the NHSBSP, screening is carried out by 103 local breast screening units. Most are based at multi-health district level and offer screening to target populations of women (aged 50–64) which number between 41 500 (a Forrest Unit) and 120 000. These units operate under the control of Quality Assurance Reference Centres, of which there is one in each region, and these are ultimately coordinated by the National Screening Coordinator, currently Mrs Julietta Patnick.

Is screening worthwhile?

Screening is a complex process with potential disadvantages for women who undertake it as well as advantages. If screening is not high quality the disadvantages may out weigh the benefits. The screening operates to tight Quality Assurance (QA) targets (Table 8.3) (Patnick 1996). QA measures need to cover every

Table 8.3 Core quality assurance targets for screening women aged 50–64 in the UK; 1994–5 results

	Target first screen	1994–5 result	Target further screens	1994–5 result
Uptake rate first invitation	70%	74.9%	N/A	89.2%
Recall rate	<7%	7.2%	<5%	3.4%
Biopsy rate	<1%	0.69%	<1%	0.36%
Cancer detection rate per 1000	>5.5	5.9	>3.5	4.3
In situ rate	10–20%	19%	10–20%	19%
Invasive cancers <15 mm	>50%	52.8%	>50%	55%

aspect of the screening programme, from maintenance of the X-ray machines, through the accuracy of mammography and cytology, to the psychological support for women undergoing screening and the acceptability to women of the programme.

Benefits and adverse effects of breast screening

The crucial benefit to be gained from the breast screening programme is reduction in deaths from breast cancer. The debate around screening hinges on the size of this mortality reduction in different groups of women, how it is affected by the method of screening, and the costs of achieving it, both human and economic. As well as a reduction in mortality, which is unequivocally achievable with a high-quality screening programme for women aged 50 and over, there are also lesser benefits in less radical treatment for women with early tumours and reassurance for women whose test results are negative (Table 8.4).

One of the major drawbacks of screening is the anxiety generated, particularly in healthy women. There is raised anxiety in the short term around the invitations for screening and the screening process itself as the woman is made aware of the possibility that she could have cancer unknowingly. For those women who are recalled from screening, there is intense short-term anxiety and distress and evidence varies as to whether this is maintained in the months after screening in women not found to have cancer (Austoker 1997). It is difficult to see how anxiety about the

Table 8.4   Benefits and disadvantages of breast screening

Benefits
   Reduced risk of dying from breast cancer for many cases detected by screening
   Less radical treatment for some early cases
   Reassurance for those with a negative screen
Disadvantages
   Pain and discomfort of mammography
   Anxiety and sometimes morbidity for those with false positive results
   False reassurance for those with false negative results
   Overdiagnosis of borderline abnormalities
   Longer to live with a cancer diagnosis for those whose prognosis is unchanged
   Radiation hazard
   Economic cost

---

screening process and results can be avoided when all the women who are involved in it know that the point of screening is a search for cancer.

The potential adverse effects of ionizing radiation used in mammography are small. At worst, the risk of developing breast cancer as a result of undergoing mammography has been calculated as one chance in a million with a latent period of 10 years. This risk is age related and lower for older women. It approaches zero within the screening age-group.

The majority of women undergoing mammography do experience discomfort (81%). 46% classify the feeling as pain and for 7% this is severe. For the great majority, however, it is short lived and bearable (McIlwaine 1993).

The potential harm from false reassurance for those whose mammograms are negative in the presence of a cancer is extremely difficult to quantify. The literature sent with the screening invitation advises women to seek help for symptoms even though their mammogram may have been negative, emphasizing that mammography does not pick up all cancers. Nevertheless, for those women who present with an interval cancer within months or a year or two of a normal screening mammogram, there may be anger and frustration, and they may wonder whether the screening process has missed their cancer (*Lancet* 1998).

Screening and subsequent assessment tests are unable to differentiate between cancer and benign disease in all cases. There will inevitably be some women who are advised to have surgical biopsies for lesions appearing suspicious at assessment but which subsequently are found to be benign. With greater use of cytology and core biopsy, the numbers of such women have been reduced. Numbers tend to be higher at the prevalent (first) screen (1.28 benign biopsies per 1000 women screened, compared with cancer detection of 5.9 per 1000 women screened 1996) than at the incident (subsequent) screen (0.08 benign biopsies per 1000 women screened, compared with 4.3 cancers detected per 1000 women screened 1996) (Patnick 1996). These women have had the distress of a possible cancer diagnosis and morbidity from unnecessary surgery for a lesion which they would have been almost certainly unaware of without screening.

Recent screening trials have found a higher incidence of breast cancer in the screened population than the control population with a cumulative excess of 10–21% in the screening population. This suggests that some questionable histological lesions may be overdiagnosed. Recent results from the Swedish Two County Study (Tabar *et al.* 1992) and the Finnish National Breast Screening Programme (Hakama *et al.* 1995) suggest that overdiagnosis is limited to the first mammographic examination. Other studies have failed to show overdiagnosis.

Allowing for the mortality reduction of between 20 and 39% in the population offered screening, there will be many women with breast cancer, even that detected on screening, who will still die of their disease. For these women screening has not altered their overall prognosis but may bring forward the time of their diagnosis thus giving them longer to live with the knowledge of their disease. At the moment there is no way of identifying these women at the time of diagnosis, and those who conduct screening know that they will only benefit a proportion of women with screen-detected cancers.

Finally, screening costs money as well as time and other resources. The average cost of screening mammography is £23.47 (Wald *et al.* 1995). Breast screening costs £23 600 per life saved. These costs have to be set against other needs within the Health Service.

Woman's decision—breast screening yes or no?

Publicity—mass media and health promotion literature (Fig. 8.3)

Most women will have heard something about breast screening in the mass media before they receive their own invitation for mammography. Messages in the news can be mixed or misleading. In health matters, a scare story will grab more attention than reiteration of the positive aspects of screening. For instance, a front page story in the *Sunday Times* in June 1991 was headlined 'Breast Cancer Screening Increases Cancer Risks For Women.' This caused women throughout the UK to cancel their appointments for screening and many who did so will not have been aware that the story which was based on unpublished Canadian Research was soon challenged in the *Sunday Times'* own letter columns and then in the *Lancet*. In contrast to the often adverse representations of screening in the newspapers, there is widespread

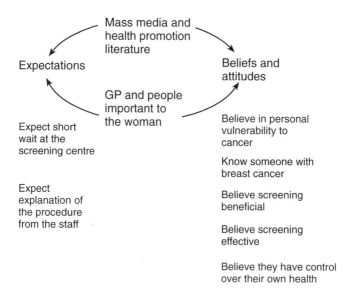

Fig. 8.3 Influences on decision to come for screening 1. Beliefs and expectations that encourage a woman to take up a screening invitation.

positive coverage of issues around screening and breast cancer in women's magazines and on television. There is no doubt that raising a woman's cancer awareness and also her own feeling of vulnerability to breast cancer will encourage her to attend for screening when offered it, but may also raise her level of anxiety about the screening process. Part of the problem with coverage about breast cancer issues in the mass media is that anxiety may be raised inappropriately, particularly in younger women who may perceive themselves to be at much higher risk of breast cancer than they actually are and who are not eligible for screening.

The invitation for screening

Once a woman reaches the age of 50 she will be offered screening the next time her doctor's practice is being screened. This will be at some stage between her fiftieth and fifty-third birthday. She may well receive encouragement from health promotion literature in the form of posters and displays in her doctor's surgery, or leaflets with the invitation for screening itself. It is important that literature offered about screening gives factual information and is honest so as to allow a woman to make an informed choice about whether to attend for screening.

It is essential that there is an explanation near the beginning of the screening process of both the benefits to be expected from screening and also the possibility of false positives and false negatives. If carefully explained this should not deter women from coming for screening. Failure to explain this may lead to a false sense of reassurance which may delay presentation of a subsequent clinical interval cancer. It may also lead to anger and frustration with the screening process for a women who suffers an interval cancer. As an editorial in the *Lancet* commented regarding cervical screening:

'If screened people are not adequately informed about the possibility of a false-negative result, it is little wonder that, when they get such a result, their next port of call is a lawyer. By that stage, they will not be interested in the distinction between a less than perfect test and less than perfect provision of a testing service'. (*Lancet* 1998).

Factors which positively influence a woman's decision to attend for screening

The charts (Figs 8.4 and 8.5) detail those factors known to influence the acceptance of the screening invitation. Some are simple

Increased likelihood of coming for screening	Decreased likelihood of coming for screening
Married	Single/divorced
Owner occupier	Urban dweller
Rural/suburban dweller	
Previous cervical smear	Longstanding illness and/or perceived poor health
Regular dental check ups	

Fig. 8.4 Influences on decision to come for screening 2. Sociodemographic factors, health status, and previous behaviour.

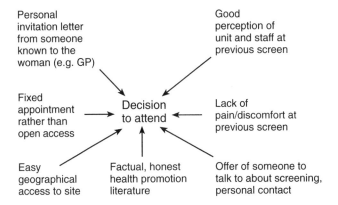

Fig. 8.5 Organizational influences on the decision to attend for screening—factors increasing the chance that a woman will accept a screening invitation.

and would appear self evident, such as the idea that a personalized letter is better than an anonymous one, that a fixed appointment is more likely to be taken up than open access, and that the harder the programme tries the greater the uptake. There are a number of factors that will predict the women that are likely to attend, for instance their expectation of the screening process and their previous uptake of other screening such as dental check ups and cervical smears. Important influences also come from other people around the woman, such as her husband and children and her GP (Majeed *et al.* 1995). A positive attitude to the consequences of breast screening, a belief that it is effective, and a perception of her own vulnerability to breast cancer are among the most important factors predicting that a woman will accept an invitation. Not surprisingly reattendance for a subsequent round of screening is also markedly influenced by the perception of the first experience of screening and the discomfort experienced at that time. (Austoker 1997; Patnick 1996).

The consequences of a woman's decision to have screening

The decision to come for screening is the most important decision that a woman will make about the screening process. It is only if she decides to come and be screened that she will have further

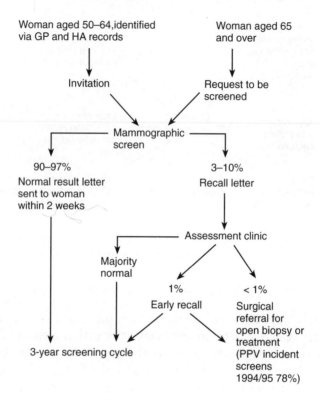

Fig. 8.6   The screening process.

involvement with the process and potential further decisions to make. Within the NHSBSP, overall acceptance within the target age-group was 72% in 1993/94 and 76.7% in 1994/95 (Patnick 1996).

Once a woman has been screened, further contacts with the screening service will be made (Fig. 8.6). For over 90% they will receive a negative result letter which will tell them that no evidence of cancer has been found (this does not exclude benign disease), that they should be aware of symptoms as screening does not detect 100% of cancers, and that they will be re-invited or have access to the programme every three years. A smaller number of women will receive a recall letter asking them to come back for assessment and further tests. For them there are other decisions to be made around screening.

A recall letter—what a woman can expect

Recall for assessment understandably causes significant adverse psychological consequences of anxiety and depression. Many recalled women react as if they have already been told that they have cancer. The majority of them will be found to be normal at further assessment (Ong and Austoker 1997). There is no doubt that a recall from screening causes distress. However, several studies assessing psychological morbidity weeks and months after a recall to assessment in women who were subsequently found to be normal (false positive) show a rapid reduction in anxiety and depression once women have been told their normal result. Bull and Campbell (1991) showed no evidence of a persisting increase in anxiety or depression six weeks following the clinic visit, indeed if anything, there was a decrease in anxiety and depression at that point, with women feeling less anxious about having breast cancer following their experience of screening and assessment. One should not, however, underestimate the anxiety felt at the time of assessment and while waiting for the assessment clinic attendance. Gram *et al.* (1990) in a study in Norway report:

'False positive mammogram was described by seven (5%) of the women as the worse thing they had ever experienced. However, most women with a false positive result regard this experience in retrospect as but one of many minor stressful experiences creating a temporary decrease in quality of life. They report the same quality of life today as women with negative screening results and 98% would attend another screening'.

In this study women were being questioned six months after their screening recall. Despite the anxiety around screening recall, very few women make the decision not to attend the assessment clinic (personal experience less than 1%).

Screening decisions—the radiologist's viewpoint

Screening differs from most other radiological subspecialities in that the radiologist is often the primary clinician dealing with the screened woman and the one who not only makes the diagnosis but breaks it to the patient. Not all radiologists are comfortable with this high level of emotional contact and there is currently a national shortage of radiologists wishing to specialize in breast screening. Another major difference between breast screening and much of the rest of radiology is that screening involves dealing with a well population. Screening radiologists therefore need to bear in mind the twin goals of not only detecting as many early cancers as possible (raising the sensitivity of the screen) but also minimizing harm through the screening process to the general population (maintaining high specificity with a low level of false positives). Maintaining the balance in the trade off between sensitivity and specificity requires radiologists working in screening to keep themselves aware of current views on the best methods of screening. Evidence, for instance, is beginning to emerge that the use of two views at all rounds of screening and more than one reader for each examination will raise the accuracy of screening. Individual radiologists may not have the resources to implement changes in the screening method in their own units but they can certainly ensure that they maintain pressure on their health authorities to keep them aware of best practice in screening and to persuade them to provide sufficient resources for a screening unit to function well (Blanks *et al.* 1998).

Radiologists and film reading

For each woman's mammogram that is read the radiologist will need to make a decision between recall or no recall. In the majority of cases the film will be clearly normal or clearly abnormal and the decision is not difficult. However, reading mammograms is an art and the distinction between subtle abnormalities and subtle variations of normal is not always easy. Recalling every woman whose mammogram shows a potential subtle abnormality will result in a high recall rate and equally, dismissing everything that is not obvious, will result in small subtle cancers being missed. These are the ones that may have most prognostic significance in terms of early detection. For an individual radiologist the decision may be made easier by arbitrating with a second reader over difficult cases. Radiologists who are working single handed do not have this option. Radiologists can hone their abilities by making sure that they always see the outcome in those cases they have recalled and use it as a learning experience. It is also helpful for them to monitor their own recall rate as comparison with national targets, and colleagues will quickly reveal if one is recalling too many or too few cases. The disadvantage of an excessively high recall rate is the distress caused to the greater number of women who are recalled for assessment and the waste of resources in assessing large numbers of women.

What happens at the assessment clinic?

An assessment clinic is staffed by a multidisciplinary team which will include a doctor (usually a radiologist, sometimes a breast clinician or a surgeon), a breast care nurse, radiographers, and clerical staff. Most women coming to assessment will be shown their mammograms and given an explanation of what the query is on their mammogram and why they have been recalled (Fig. 8.7).

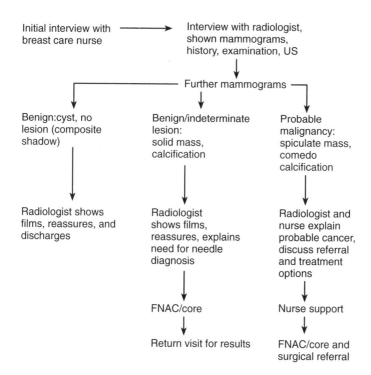

Fig. 8.7   Assessment procedures at south west London Breast Screening Service.

They will also be told what to expect during the clinic visit. Subsequently a history will be taken, clinical examination carried out, further imaging (ultrasound and any further mammography) performed, and if necessary needle biopsies (cytology, cyst aspiration, or core biopsy) will also be done, often on the same visit. At the end of this process women can expect a further interview with the doctor to discuss the findings of the clinic visit and give them an indication of whether the findings are benign or malignant. When cytology or core biopsy has been taken, women may need to return for a second visit to be given the results of these tests. For many women the original mammographic abnormality will turn out to have been simply a composite shadow or asymmetric tissue, they can be reassured that no genuine lesion is present and discharged back to the routine screening programme with no further choices to make.

The radiologist and assessment

At an assessment clinic it is the radiologist's task to determine whether a woman has a probable cancer or not, while simultaneously informing the woman throughout the clinic process what is happening and, when necessary, sympathetically breaking bad news. In our clinic a breast care nurse will be the first point of contact. She explains to women what will happen at the clinic, assesses their emotional state, and encourages them, if they wish, to bring their companion with them during their interview with the doctor. For those women found to have a probable malignancy the breast care nurse will also be the last point of contact at the clinic and will provide continuing support afterwards.

The radiologists will then see the woman to show her films and explain in simple terms why she has been recalled (e.g. a density on the mammogram which is different from the previous screening film) and what needs to be done at the clinic. The radiologist will also take a history, examine the woman, and perform ultrasound where needed. At the end of this the radiologist should be able to give the woman an idea of their findings so far (e.g. that there is a lump to feel in the breast which also shows up on the ultrasound). They will then arrange for the woman to have any further mammographic views. The purpose of this initial discussion is for the radiologist to gain the information required from the history, examination, and ultrasound, while conveying to the woman what is happening, what she can expect from the clinic, and that she can expect some sort of a result by the end of the clinic. I personally do not mention the word cancer in this first interview. Most women come into an assessment clinic in a state of marked anxiety. The knowledge that they will get some sort of an answer that day at the end of their visit but not immediately during the current interview allows their anxiety to reduce a little and permits them to start taking in information.

While she is having her extra mammographic views, a woman has a little time to start digesting the information she has already been given. Once the further mammographic views have been taken the radiologist should be in a position to determine whether the lesion which originally prompted recall is clearly benign (e.g. a cyst or positional shadow), and the woman can at this point be told that she is clear of cancer and discharged. Alternatively the lesion may be clearly malignant or indeterminate/probably benign.

Women with probably benign lesions

These are usually woman who have either indeterminate-/benign-appearing calcifications or a solid mass which appears benign on imaging and is probably a fibroadenoma. Both these findings are common in the screening programme. The radiologist at this point needs to show the woman all her imaging and explain, usually with the aid of diagrams, exactly why he/she feels the lesion is unlikely to be a cancer, at the same time explaining a need for cytology or core biopsy to confirm this. The results of these tests will usually not be available at the same clinic, so the woman will need to return at another date for her results. In the majority of cases the results of the tissue examination will be benign and the woman can then be either discharged to routine screening or placed on early recall to be sure of stability before discharge. In some cases, however, the procedure will reveal unexpected malignancy (PPV (positive predictive value) for indeterminate calcifications in South West London approximately 20%, PPV for round, benign-appearing masses approximately 2%). The radiologist needs to tread a delicate line when talking to these women at the assessment clinic, providing enough reassurance so that when the needle test confirms a benign result the woman is content to accept follow-up or discharge, but not reassuring so heavily that the woman thinks there is no possibility of a malignant outcome and would find it shocking.

The woman's perspective on a benign outcome

The majority of women are satisfied with the benign diagnosis. A small number of women, however, (in our unit less than 1%) are worried by the idea of a breast lesion even if they are asymptomatic and have been reassured of its benignity and will opt for surgery. In addition, early recall can lead to raised anxiety. Brown *et al.* (1997) found that 3 out of 191 women in an early follow-up group failed to re-attend because of anxiety. Some women, however, in our experience indicate that they find it reassuring to be placed on early recall; they like the idea that someone is keeping an eye on them. They also have a contact number at the unit for advice if they have queries. Usually early recall is only used once for probably benign lesions to ensure stability before discharge back to the routine screening programme.

Women with highly suspicious lesions at assessment

Less than 1% of screened women will be found to have a lesion at assessment that is strongly suspicious or diagnostic of malignancy, and referral for surgical biopsy and treatment will be recommended. When the results of assessment indicate that a lesion is strongly suspicious of a carcinoma, the radiologists will need to break this news to a woman during their second interview following further mammographic views. The radiologist will usually have built up to this point with a hierarchy of information during the clinic (e.g. a density on the mammogram when a woman first arrives becomes a lump which can be felt on clinical examination, and a dense lump on the ultrasound, then, a likely cancer following the further mammographic views). Having built up to the point of diagnosis it is important that the word cancer is spoken as otherwise a woman can go away from an assessment clinic with a referral to a surgeon still not being sure whether she is being told that her lesion is malignant or not. As well as getting this essential message across, it is important that the radiologist assesses each individual woman's capacity to take in information.

A woman who has been assessed following routine screening enters the clinic as a well woman and usually has very little knowledge about breast cancer and what will happen to her following the assessment clinic. It is a demanding task for the radiologist to get across enough information for a woman who, at this point, is usually in shock to enable her to make informed decisions about whether to accept referral onto a surgeon, which surgeon or hospital she would like to go to, and to begin to think about what sort of treatment she would like. In addition at this point, although the majority of women referred on for surgery will have cancer, some of these suspicious lesions will turn out to be benign and the radiologist still needs to make sure that a woman is aware that only a tissue diagnosis can provide 100% confirmation of malignancy. Also, the majority of screen-detected cancers will be either *in situ* or small tumours less than 15 mm in diameter. There is therefore a balance of optimism and pessimism to be conveyed to the woman. She needs to know that there is still a possibility that her lesion is benign and also a probability in many cases that it will carry a good prognosis.

The presence of a relative or friend, where the woman wishes it, is often helpful as they provide a second pair of ears to take in information. In addition it is extremely helpful to have breast care nurse support during this interview. The radiologist is the person who breaks the bad news but the nurse can provide support after the interview with the doctor. The presence of the nurse listening and asking open questions in a calm unhurried way often allows the woman to express fears or concern which she did not wish to 'bother the doctor' with.

For women with a cancer diagnosis the assessment clinic is their first opportunity to find out about their disease and make choices about their management. They are unlikely to remember many facts after this interview with the radiologist so it is important that the doctor ensures that they have retained some key messages (e.g. that this is a probable cancer diagnosis, where appropriate that the prognosis is good, when and where they will see the surgeon) and that they have a contact telephone number and name for further information and support.

Assessment—malignant outcome—the woman's perspective

For these women their worst fears around screening have been realized. By this stage a woman is often expecting to be told she has cancer. It is essential when talking about a lesion that a woman sees her films and has them explained to her. Even when the abnormality is a cancer, the actual size of it on the mammogram is often much less than in the woman's imagination and seeing the films is reassuring.

Women have very varied reactions to being given a probable cancer diagnosis. For some women who have found the extreme uncertainty of the recall and assessment process unbearable, being told that they probably do have cancer is paradoxically almost a relief as they can start on the first stage of dealing with it. For others this is the worst moment of their lives, although they may keep their emotions under control until a later point. Women's fears around a cancer diagnosis are also very varied. For some the greatest fear is the thought of death or mutilating surgery. Others are frightened of adjuvant treatment such as chemotherapy, and for many it is practical considerations such as who will look after their dog while they are in hospital, or who will care for a disabled husband or elderly relative, or how they will tell their family about their diagnosis. An unhurried interview and the asking of open questions gives an opportunity for a woman to express herself and to voice her fears. It is always tempting for the doctor giving a cancer diagnosis to rush in with immediate reassurance, but this may stifle the opportunity for a woman to ask questions about the things that bother her most.

The whole visit to the assessment clinic and particularly this interview are distressing, and the way in which the news is broken to a woman may colour her whole feelings about the treatment of her cancer. A woman is likely to be shocked and unable to take in more than a limited amount of information at this point of first diagnosis, the person accompanying her may well be able to take in more information and think more clearly.

There are a number of decisions to be made at this point. Firstly the woman must decide whether she accepts referral onwards for treatment. A few women, in our experience less than 0.5% of these offered referral, will refuse treatment. Interestingly they usually accept further follow-up in the screening unit and often change their minds and decide to opt for surgery at a later visit when the uncertainty and anxiety of continued follow-up comes home to them. Most women, however, wish to press on as fast as possible with referral to a surgeon. They may need to make choices about which surgeon or hospital they go to. They may be influenced by the reputation of a particular hospital, by ease of access, or by previous experience. Women will also indicate, often non-verbally, how much information they want to receive at this point; some for instance will wish to know all about the side-effects and benefits of chemotherapy and for others it will be enough to know that there may be further treatment offered following surgery. It is important that the doctor and nurse are sensitive to verbal and non-verbal communication from the woman, and tailor the information they give to her needs.

A conclusion

Breast screening is a complex area, there are proven benefits for screened women, and there are disadvantages. I find one of the greatest challenges of screening for me personally to be the issue of conveying sufficient information to women at each stage so that they can make a truly informed choice without suffering from ignorance or information or emotion overload. Giving either too little or too much information may leave a woman confused and unable to make informed decisions about her future care.

I know that only a proportion of women with screen-detected cancers will have their lives saved by screening. Others will have less aggressive lesions which would not have progressed to kill them or will already have incurable systemic disease. Yet, in order to benefit that proportion, as many women as possible need to be encouraged to go through the screening process. They need to know what they are committing themselves to, and to be kept fully informed at each stage of screening. If women are not in a position to understand the delicate balance of advantage and disadvantage which makes up breast cancer screening, those that suffer the disadvantages (in particular false positive and false negative screens) will become angry and disillusioned with screening and make their feelings public to the detriment of the programme.

Wendy—a personal view

Four years ago I was called to have a routine mammogram because I had reached the age of 50. It did not occur to me at the time that I would be diagnosed as having breast cancer until I was recalled to the breast screening unit.

I turned up for my appointment and was called into a small room where a nurse informed me that if I had any worries at any time or doubts or questions to always ask. I was given another mammogram and an ultrasound scan. The doctor told me she was 90% certain I had a small lump the size of a pea, that it was cancerous, and that it would have to be removed. My immediate thought was that I felt fine. I am a keep fit person, play badminton, and have a fair amount of energy, so why should this make too much difference to me now?

The doctor explained the procedure for the removal of the lump, and that the breast cancer unit to which I was being referred was excellent. I would be given an appointment to see the consultant within four to six weeks. I have to say I questioned the amount of time I had to wait. I was reassured that I wasn't an urgent case, although psychologically the sooner I had the operation the better. So far the decisions regarding my breast cancer were all made for me, and that suited me personally.

Subsequent to my diagnosis I became a Breast Cancer Care volunteer and in my experience I think that women react in many different ways depending on the attitude of the patient and the manner of the doctor when she is being told she has a breast cancer diagnosis. Some patients are not able or willing to make decisions at that time because they are so frightened of the future. Patients react in many ways because of their personalities and different experiences. It must be very difficult for doctors and nurses to know whether the decisions on treatment options should be left to patients. I think it must also depend on the support the patient has from family and friends. I have had marvellous support from my husband, sons, family, and friends. I think it helped me personally to be able to talk about my breast cancer and to have a positive attitude.

Three weeks after my diagnosis I was called to the hospital to have a biopsy and my husband came with me. I felt it was very important for him to be involved. I had the results the same day. I felt very confident with the surgeon and he explained everything as it was happening. A week later I returned to the clinic and the surgeon was there with the oncologist who said he would like me to have a course of radiation treatment. He explained why this would be of benefit after my operation. They also discussed with me the removal of the lymph glands under my arm and why that would also be a good idea. They asked for my view on their suggestions and I responded by saying that they were the experts and I would do whatever was recommended. I did not want the decision to be left to me. The oncologist then asked me if I was willing to take part in a chemotherapy clinical trial. They gave me an excellent explanation about the treatment and made it clear that my life span without chemotherapy would be good and that I might not necessarily benefit from this treatment. I was given a fair amount of literature on radiotherapy and chemotherapy which I read thoroughly. Because of the amount of drugs I would have to take or have injected, I decided selfishly against having chemotherapy. I have no regrets at having made this decision.

Three weeks from diagnosis I had a lumpectomy and the lymph glands removed. I made a good recovery. The surgery was followed by radiotherapy treatment and I agreed to participate in a radiotherapy trial.

One thing I forgot to mention is the fact that when the doctor explained about tamoxifen he did outline the advantages of taking the drug for approximately five years.

9

Decision-making for breast cancer predisposition gene testing: considerations in women at risk, their relatives, and health care professionals

R.A. Eeles and A. Ardern-Jones

Background to genetic predisposition to breast cancer

Cancer is a genetic disease at the cellular level because a cancer arises when genetic changes occur in the cancer cell. In a proportion of cases, a genetic change is inherited (in the germ line) and predisposes to the other changes causing cancer development. About 5–10% of breast and ovarian cancers occur as a result of highly penetrant germ-line mutations in cancer-predisposition genes (Easton and Peto 1990; Claus *et al.* 1990; 1991). One of these genes, *BRCA1*, predisposing to breast and/or ovarian cancer, was mapped to the long arm of chromosome 17 in 1990 (Hall *et al.* 1990; Narod *et al.* 1991) and cloned (identified) in 1994 (Miki *et al.* 1994). Collaborative studies by the Breast Cancer Linkage Consortium (BCLC) have shown that *BRCA1* mutations are responsible for about 50% of families with clear dominant predisposition to breast cancer and over 80% of families segregating both breast and ovarian cancer (Easton *et al.* 1993; Ford *et al.* 1998). A majority (32% of the total; Ford *et al.* 1998) of the remaining high-risk breast cancer families, including most families segregating both male and female breast cancer (76% of these), are due to a second predisposition gene, *BRCA2*, on chromosome 13, which was cloned in 1995 (Wooster *et al.* 1995).

Studies by the BCLC have provided estimates of the cancer risks in carriers of mutations in *BRCA1* and these figures can be used in counselling (Easton *et al.* 1993; 1995; Ford *et al.* 1994; 1998). Based on the incidence of disease in *BRCA1* families, Easton *et al.* (1995) estimated the risk of breast cancer to be 51% by age 50 and 85% by age 70. These high risks have been confirmed by studying the risk of contralateral breast cancer in gene carriers who have already developed one cancer (Ford *et al.* 1994), and by a study of a large Utah kindred (Goldgar *et al.* 1994). The risk of ovarian cancer has been estimated to be 63% by age 70, based on the ovarian cancer incidence in *BRCA1* families or 44% based on the risk of ovarian cancer in carriers with a previous breast cancer (Easton *et al.* 1995). There is some evidence that the ovarian cancer risk is mutation dependent (Easton *et al.* 1995). Gayther *et al.* (1995) have found that mutations towards the 5′ end (the beginning) of *BRCA1* confer a higher risk of ovarian cancer than those towards the 3′ end, a result also found by Holt *et al.* (1996). In our opinion, the best risk estimates for counselling purposes at the present time are those derived from the BCLC studies, i.e. a lifetime risk of ovarian cancer of 63%, ignoring the possibility of allelic heterogeneity (the fact that different mutations may have different risks). This situation may change, however, if the evidence of allelic heterogeneity becomes stronger. The risk of ovarian cancer in *BRCA2* is also raised (27% by age 80) but is not as high as for *BRCA1* (Ford *et al.* 1998). The population risk is just below 1%.

There is also some evidence of increased risks of colon and prostate cancer in *BRCA1* gene carriers. At least two *BRCA1* families are known to contain male breast cancer cases but the risk appears to be substantially lower than for *BRCA2*. *BRCA2* carries a 5% risk of male breast cancer. The risk of colon cancer in *BRCA1* is estimated to be increased four-fold, and the risk of prostate cancer is estimated to be increased three-fold, corresponding to an absolute risk for each cancer of about 6% by age 70 (Ford *et al.* 1994); in *BRCA2* the prostate cancer risk is 6–14% by age 70 (BCLC data).

The carrier frequency of *BRCA1* mutations in the general population of the UK has been estimated indirectly from epidemiological studies at about 1 in 800 people, with the range of plausible estimates being 1 in 500 to 1 in 2500 (Ford

Table 9.1 Proportion of single cases due to *BRCA1* by age estimated from the gene frequency

Age	Breast cancer cases (%)	Ovarian cancer cases (%)
20–29	7.5	5.9
30–39	5.1	5.6
40–49	2.2	4.6
50–59	1.4	2.6
60–69	0.8	1.8
20–69	1.7	2.8

Source: From Ford *et al*. 1995

et al. 1995). The corresponding estimated frequencies amongst breast and ovarian cancer cases at different ages are shown in Table 9.1. Studies of early onset breast cancer cases in Boston and Seattle have found *BRCA1* carrier rates which are in good agreement with these estimates (Fitzgerald *et al.* 1996; Langston *et al.* 1996). Much higher frequencies are known to apply to Ashkenazi Jews, owing to a founder effect involving mainly a particular mutation (185delAG, a deletion of two bases from the code; Struewing *et al.* 1995a). This mutation has an estimated frequency of about 1% in Ashkenazi Jews, and about 20% in Jewish women diagnosed with breast cancer under 40 (Struewing *et al.* 1995a; Offit *et al.* 1996; Roa *et al.* 1996). This rises to 67% in families with breast and ovarian cancer (Tonin *et al.* 1996). There is another mutation in *BRCA1* which is more commonly seen in Ashkenazis and another in *BRCA2* (6174delT, a deletion of one base from the code) which is present in 1.5% of this population (Neuhausen *et al.* 1996; Oddoux *et al.* 1996).

Prior to the cloning of *BRCA1*, predictive genetic testing was possible by linkage analysis, which is the analysis of the inheritance of the genetic areas (markers) around the area within which the *BRCA1* gene lies. Multiple samples from extensive families are needed for such an analysis and only a limited number of families in the UK had enough affected individuals sampled to be able to be offered this test. The problem with testing by linkage is that it has a degree of uncertainty because there is only a certain prior probability that the gene is running in the family. The advantages of the cloning of *BRCA1* are that more individuals

Table 9.2 Threshold for probability of *BRCA1/2* mutation

Chance that a mutation is present[a]	Clinical criteria
<10%	All single cases of breast of ovarian cancer
10%	Single breast cancer cases <35 years
⩾20%	⩾2 breast cancer cases <50 years
	1 breast cancer <40 years in an Ashkenazi
⩾20%–⩽50%	3 breast cancer cases <50 years
	4–5 breast cancer cases, no ovarian
	1 breast and 1 ovarian cancer
>50%	>1 breast and >1 ovarian cancer
	⩾4 cases of female/male breast cancer
	6+ female cases of breast cancer

Source: Langston *et al.* 1996; Franks *et al.* 1997; Ford *et al.* 1998.
[a] The chance of *detecting* a mutation is lower because:
At least 15% of mutations are regulatory, i.e. are not in the coding region of the gene which is the area tested.
The genetic screening methods to find the mutation initially are about 80% sensitive (the test, once the mutation is known is very accurate—≈0.04% error rate).

will be able to be tested because the mutation has to be confirmed in a smaller number of affected family members than for linkage analysis. Once the mutation is found, the test is also more accurate. The dilemma is at what threshold prior probability should *BRCA1* testing be offered. *BRCA2* testing in the UK is much more in its infancy and is only available on a research basis. Estimates of the prior probabilities of families being due to germ line mutations in *BRCA1/2* are shown in Table 9.2. As a summary statement, if a threshold prior probability of the presence of a *BRCA1* mutation of 10% is used, this would exclude the testing of all single cases of breast cancer over 35 years or ovarian cancer at any age, with the exception of the Ashkenazi Jewish population. A threshold of 10% would involve the testing of families with two or more cases of breast cancer diagnosed at less than 50 years or two ovarian cancers at less than 60 years. In practice, most centres may have to limit testing to a higher threshold of ⩾50% chance of a *BRCA1/2* mutation. This would be limited to clusters of at least four cases of breast cancer at <60 years/ ovarian cancer at any age.

The process of genetic testing

The counselling process for individuals considering genetic testing should involve an explanation of the nature of genetic inheritance and the fact that the specific alteration has to be found in the family first in order to offer an unaffected person a test, so that if it is negative then this is truly a negative result. A lot of individuals do not appreciate this and think that testing involves the taking of a blood sample and the availability of a result in a few days. They also do not appreciate that if a result in this situation is negative, that it does not exclude that they have a breast cancer predisposition gene, as the mutation in the family has not been identified first. The reporting of genetic testing in the media has simplified the genetic testing process which has confounded this misunderstanding.

The current suggested protocols are modelled on those for Huntington's disease, namely at least two counselling sessions which, in the UK, are at least one month apart (the 'cooling off' period), although in some US series these were only a day apart (Lerman *et al.* 1996). Results should, if possible, be given to individuals face-to-face in the presence of a supportive relative or friend.

All testing should explain the psychosocial and insurance implications. Currently, any results of a genetic test have to be declared when applying for a new insurance policy. Some policies may be exempt from this declaration if the Association of British Insurers Moratorium for life cover for mortgages of $<£100,000$ is extended in 1999.

Summary

- Only 5–10% of breast cancers occur in individuals with a breast cancer predisposition gene.
- Of these, 5–10%, about half are due to *BRCA1/2*, so further genes remain to be discovered.
- Affected individuals have to be tested *first* to identify the mutation in the family so that a negative test in unaffecteds is truly negative.

- Due to founder effects, the Ashkenazi population has a higher chance of having specific mutations.
- Lifetime (by age 80) cancer risks in carriers:

Gene	Cancer type (%)				
	Female breast	Ovarian	Male breast	Colon	Prostate[a]
BRCA1	80–85[b]	60	?0 approx.	6	6
BRCA2	80–85	27	5	?0	6–14

[a] By age 74
[b] This may be lower in Ashkenazis (~ 36–60%)

Decision-making processes in individuals undergoing predictive genetic testing, their relatives, and health care professionals

From the preceding background, it can be deduced that the following factors weigh in decision-making in these respective groups.

1. Individuals considering testing (the 'testee')

The need to know
The ending of uncertainty is a significant factor for many people considering genetic testing (Craufurd *et al.* 1989). In studies of families in a research setting offered *BRCA1* testing by linkage, the need to end uncertainty was the third reason given in a list of order of importance for having the test (Watson *et al.* 1995; 1996). In Huntington's disease, where the knowledge that one has the gene means a certainty of developing early-onset dementia, the ending of uncertainty was a major factor for taking the test (Evers-Kiebooms *et al.* 1996). Evers-Kiebooms *et al.* (1997) have shown that there is no increased psychological morbidity from knowledge of genetic status, even in those who proved to be carriers of Huntington's disease at five years after the test is performed.

Knowledge of cancer risks
Genetic testing, if negative, can reduce individuals' risks to those of the general population if the mutation has already been found

in the family. Even in those who are found to carry a mutation in whom the cancer risk is known to be high, it is emphasized in the counselling process that this is not always 100% for all cancer predisposition genes. In particular, for the breast cancer predisposition genes *BRCA1* and *BRCA2*, the breast cancer risk is 85% and not 100% by the age of 80. At present, we do not know the other factors which may interact with genetic status to cause breast cancer, and studies are in progress to determine what they might be.

The higher probabilities that a breast cancer predisposition gene is present in certain ethnic groups such as Ashkenazis may not be realized until counselled.

Uptake of the test and reaction to the results
Results of the uptake and reasons for testing in *BRCA1*-linked families showed that the test has a higher uptake in women (Craufurd *et al.* 1995; Watson *et al.* 1995). The uptake in these studies has been much higher (about 60%) than that described for Huntington's disease (16%; Craufurd *et al.* 1989). However, these results are from small numbers of individuals and they were mainly in families which had taken part in research programmes and which may be very highly motivated to take the test. The main reason for testing was for the children of those tested (Watson *et al.* 1995). Interestingly, in Watson's study, a proportion of women thought that having the test would stop the disease, despite having had two sessions of genetic counselling to explain that testing merely alters the level of risk but does not determine exactly if or when the disease will develop. Studies of the perception of risk have shown that individuals' personal perception of risk is not related to the absolute value, but is related to the risk perception process (Marteau *et al.* 1991; Struewing *et al.* 1995b). This may be altered by the cancer burden in the family—the so-called 'cancer legacy' (Ardern-Jones 1997). Women are more likely than men to undertake genetic testing, despite having the same chance of having inherited the gene (Lerman *et al.* 1996; Watson *et al.* 1996). This may be because women are more likely to take up health prevention measures.

There has been much concern that insurance issues will influence test uptake; in our series this has not been found to be the case to date (Watson *et al.* 1996), but a larger analysis is needed. In the USA it was a factor for 16% of testees (Lerman *et al.* 1996).

The personality and risk perception in the individual undergoing testing is important in their reaction to test results. Those who believe themselves to be at high risk expect positive results and cope better than those who believe they will get a negative test results and then are subsequently found to be positive (Lynch *et al.* 1993). Our results at one year follow-up did not show psychological morbidity from testing but numbers were small (Watson *et al.* 1996). The uptake of testing and the effect on psychological morbidity and cancer anxiety is being studied in a large multicentre study in the UK (coordinators M. Watson, R. Eeles, and G. Evans; funded by the Cancer Research Campaign).

The uptake of the test in relation to treatment
Uptake for DNA testing is much higher for conditions for which there is treatment. Uptake is higher in breast cancer predisposition than Huntington's disease and is even higher (80%) for familial adenomatous polyposis for which there is effective treatment (Evans *et al.* 1997). The genetic test result can alter management; for example, if a woman would like a prophylactic mastectomy if she had a breast cancer predisposition gene but would uptake screening if a test could not be offered, then a counsellee may decide to uptake genetic testing to help in decision-making for prevention. 50% of *BRCA* gene carriers in one UK study decided to have prophylactic mastectomy (Lalloo *et al.* 1998); however, in some American studies the prophylactic mastectomy uptake rate is as low as 17% (Lerman *et al.* 1996). The cause for the low uptake rates in the US is unknown but may be due to insurance issues because some insurance companies will not pay for prophylactic surgery.

2. *The impact of genetic testing on the testees' relatives*

Inherited diseases, by definition, may or may not affect other family members. In this respect they are different from other diseases and the family, in this context, may be regarded as the patient. The new and developing area of cancer genetics may have serious implications for family members and Nelkin (1992) warns of a new 'genetic underclass' or 'the presymptomatic ill'. Therefore, it is essential for families to be fully aware of all the possible implications with regard to any genetic testing.

Research involving families coping with cancer highlights the adjustments and problems that exist for all family members (Lewis 1986; Northouse 1988). While cancer is a common disease, there is inevitably an association of cancer as a life-threatening illness. This is compounded by the public perception of cancer as a 'Killer Disease' (Sontag 1991; Daily Mail 1997). Therefore in a culture of wellness, cancer may bring some families together or, in contrast, may pull them apart. Indeed, no families escape change as a result of a cancer diagnosis.

The experience of several close family members who have died of cancer and, more importantly, how they have died may be perceived as a 'cancer legacy' and may introduce imbalance into normal family relationships (Weihs and Reiss 1996). In a cancer family with a hereditary predisposition this can be a real experience with many complex bereavement issues. Many families lose their relatives at a very young age and the cancer-related losses, with painful maladaptive changes, may increase the feelings of fear and anxiety regarding cancer within the family. Uncertainty linked to psychological morbidity may become unmanageable without the support of the family or the health professional.

Families attending the Cancer Genetics Clinic need to be assured of a confidential genetic counselling service. The subjects of cancer genes and modes of inheritance are difficult for most people to understand and therefore any family stories must be taken seriously by the health professionals (Blaxter 1983; Cornwell 1984; Richards 1996; Ardern-Jones 1997). Thus, health professionals working in this area must be aware that the scientific paradigm of health practice and 'folk' concepts may be in opposition and need clarification.

Indeed, McGuire (1979) found that people with a hereditary risk of malignant melanoma appreciated simple reassurance and consideration from the health professional and regarded this as therapeutic. Feelings of guilt, isolation and depression are often cited as part of being in a family with a hereditary condition (Burton 1975). The significance of support is essential from a nursing perspective and nurse researchers Mahon and Caspeson (1995) found that family members with a hereditary cancer predisposition very often felt isolated and misunderstood. Therefore, by promoting subjectivity and allowing insight into another person the philosopher Heidegger (1962) interpreted this understanding as caring. Benner and Wrubel (1989) argue that Heidegger's model for caring should underpin all professional nursing care and the focus should therefore be on understanding from the patient's perspective, his/her perceptions and beliefs. It is of considerable value for all health professionals working in the rapidly developing area of cancer genetics to spend time listening to the complex stories of family members (Ardern-Jones 1997).

Time in a nurse-led clinic in the genetic testing programme should be made available, both for family members wishing to be tested and for those who prefer to take further time to consider whether testing is the right option for them. Indeed, in such a clinic, the client needs to understand fully the risks and benefits of testing, thus balancing scientific knowledge with his/her personal feelings and beliefs that make sense to his/her way of living in the world. The trained cancer nurse involved in this important caring role needs to have a thorough knowledge of cancer genetics, combined with the skill and art of nursing and the ability to clarify issues that may need to be untangled from a legacy of family stories.

Inter-family relationships can be complicated by the testing process. Relatives who may not have had contact for many years can find it difficult to approach an affected member of the family to take the initial blood test to identify the mutation. This may be compounded if the individual is seriously ill because the individual seeking testing may be viewed by the family as being heartless for asking a seriously ill individual to give a blood test at a time when they undergoing treatment or are near to death (France 1998). Individuals who subsequently test negative may experience survivor guilt (Huggins *et al.* 1992) or there may no longer be a close family tie of the genetic risk that previously bonded them into the family (Tibben *et al.* 1990). Close relatives (particularly partners) may be more affected if an individual tests positive than the actual carrier themselves (Lynch *et al.* 1993). The cancer burden (Lloyd *et al.* 1996) in the family (the number of cases, age at diagnosis, and experience of the illness process, in particular the age of the individual at risk when relatives have died) is very important. The mother–daughter phenomenon is well recognized (Wellisch *et al.* 1991; 1992). Wellisch *et al.* showed that women who have lost their mothers when they are in their teens are the most psychologically distressed by the experience of cancer in the family. This may impact on the uptake of testing and is currently being investigated as a subsidiary study in the UK study of predictive genetic testing (C. Foster, personal communication).

3. The decision-making process in the health care professional

Predictive genetic testing for breast cancer predisposition can influence screening measures and treatment options and alter the physician's level of vigilance of symptoms. The experience of the difference in level of screening as a result of genetic testing is not yet reported; however, if genetic testing results in a negative result then screening can sometimes be stopped. If there is gene alteration on one side of the family and the other side of the family has a level of cancer that would warrant screening and the gene alteration has not been found on that side of the family, then screening cannot always be withdrawn. However, in many cases a negative breast cancer predisposition gene test will reduce the risk to that of the general population, in which case they can be offered population screening and do not need earlier mammographic screening. We have certainly had the experience of individuals, whose test is negative, refusing to stop their screening because they feel 'safe' while they are being monitored. This is, however, anecdotal and the exact size of this problem is unknown. In our experience to date, it occurs in about 2% of individuals tested.

Genetic testing may also alter the type of treatment offered. Individuals with a mutation in a gene called *TP53* are more resistant to the killing effects of radiation; however, their cells accumulate damage in DNA. There may therefore be a risk of radiation-induced second tumours above that of the general population (Eeles 1993). *TP53* is most commonly found in classical Li-Fraumeni syndrome, which is very rare. This is the association of childhood sarcoma with early onset breast and other tumours (brain, leukaemia, adrenocortical, and sarcoma). Although it is rare, such families do warrant testing because tumours that could be managed by either radiation or surgery should be managed surgically. Furthermore, follow-up should be with imaging using non-radiological modalities.

Several cancer predisposition genes confer an increased risk of more than one type of cancer; for example, the *BRCA1/2* genes result in an increased risk of breast and ovarian cancer. Many oncologists would offer ovarian oblation as adjuvant treatment for breast cancer because it improves survival (Early Breast Cancer Trialists' Collaborative Group 1995). In individuals with a *BRCA1/2* mutation, one may offer ovarian oblation by oophorectomy rather than irradiation or Zoladex which would leave the ovaries *in situ*. Indeed, irradiation may theoretically induce further tumours, although this is not proven. There is much debate about whether to offer prostate cancer screening to male carriers.

The bar to offering more widespread testing at present is threefold. The first is technical; the screening of the *BRCA1* and *BRCA2* genes for mutations is extremely labour-intensive. *BRCA1* has 23 exons (1–24; exon 4 is missing), of which 22 code for a protein of 1863 amino acids (Miki *et al.* 1994). Over 100 distinct mutations in *BRCA1* have been described to date (Shattuck-Eidens *et al.* 1995; 1997; BIC database, accessible on the Internet at http://www.nchgr.nih.gov/dir/lab_transfer/bic/.). These mutations are widely scattered across the gene. A very similar mutation pattern occurs in *BRCA2* which is about twice as large. The vast majority of mutations have, however, so far only been observed in limited numbers of families (this is why the specific mutation has to be determined in each family prior to offering testing). Most result in a truncation (shortening) of the BRCA1 protein due to the insertion or deletion of bases in the coding sequence (frameshifts) or are nonsense mutations which convert a coding base into a stop code.

The second problem is that a small proportion of linked families (perhaps 10–20%) appear to contain no alterations in the *BRCA1* genetic code. Individuals from some of these families have been shown to express only the normal BRCA1 protein (i.e. the mechanism that tells both copies of the *BRCA* gene to work is faulty), suggesting the presence of a regulatory mutation. Thus, the absence of a *BRCA1* mutation in the coding region, even after rigorous sequencing, cannot rule out the possibility that a linked family is due to *BRCA1*. A functional test which directly measures the effect of a *BRCA1* alteration is preferable but is not yet available and there is intensive research to develop this.

The final problem is that many clusters of breast cancer are not due to *BRCA1/2* and are due to another gene or genes and these have not yet been discovered and therefore cannot be tested.

In summary, there are many factors influencing decision-making in genetic testing for predisposition to breast cancer which impact upon the individual considering testing, their relatives, and health care professionals. More research is needed in this area, particularly as more alterations are found in *BRCA1/2* in families who have not previously taken part in research studies. It is possible that research families are highly motivated to uptake testing. Breast cancer patients in the oncology clinic, who have not previously taken part in gene-finding studies, may have a much lower uptake. All testing at present should be undertaken using ethically-reviewed protocols and should be performed by cancer genetics teams in specialist units. However, as the technical difficulties associated with testing are overcome and the application of testing to oncological management increases, testing will become more widespread as part of the general oncological management of the breast cancer patient. The impact of testing on family dynamics should not be forgotten in this process and the role of the multidisciplinary team involving cancer geneticists, oncologists, psychologists, and clinical nurse specialists, will be paramount to ensure that tests are accompanied by appropriate counselling and support for the testee and their relatives.

10

Breast cancer prevention using tamoxifen

L. Assersohn and T. J. Powles

Breast cancer is the most common cancer in women in UK, with one in 12 women developing the disease at some point in their lives. Epidemiological evidence suggests that oestrogen acts as a promoter in the pathogenesis of breast cancer with factors such as early menarche, late menopause, nulliparity, and delayed first pregnancy conferring an increased risk. In addition, it is known that there is a familial tendency to develop the disease with a woman's risk especially increased if her mother or sister develop breast cancer before the age of 50. Some women have a significantly increased risk of developing breast cancer by inheriting mutations of either the *BRCA1* or *BRCA2* gene. These, and other highly penetrant genes, account for 10–12% of the breast cancers which occur.

Oestrogen is an important factor in the endocrine promotion of breast cancer. Consequently, the risk of developing breast cancer may be reduced by blocking oestrogenic activity in the breast, using an antioestrogen, such as tamoxifen, as a potential chemoprevention agent.

Why tamoxifen?

Tamoxifen is a non-steroidal triphenylethylene derivative which has both oestrogenic and antioestrogenic activities. It will inhibit the growth of oestrogen receptor-positive MCF7 cells *in vivo* (Lippman and Bolan 1975) and arrest the development of oestrogen-dependent mammary tumours in carcinogenically treated rats (Jordan 1976). Similarly, the administration of tamoxifen prevents the development of breast tumours in mice infected with the mouse mammary tumour virus (Jordan *et al.* 1990).

In the clinical setting, tamoxifen was used initially to treat postmenopausal women with metastatic breast cancer, when it was found to have low toxicity and produce remissions in approximately 30% of patients (Cole *et al.* 1971; Legha and Carter 1976; Manni *et al.* 1976; Legha *et al.* 1979). Consequently, tamoxifen was used as adjuvant therapy after primary surgery for early breast cancer and a meta-analysis of over 30 000 women treated within randomized trials (Early Breast Cancer Trialists' Collaborative Group 1992) showed that tamoxifen given for more than two years reduced the overall recurrence rates by 38% and mortality rates by 24%. In addition, it was shown that women who received two or more years of adjuvant treatment with tamoxifen had a 40% decrease in the incidence of contralateral breast cancer (Rutqvist *et al.* 1991; Early Breast Cancer Trialists' Collaborative Group 1992).

These results have encouraged the introduction of randomized controlled clinical trials to investigate the use of tamoxifen in the chemoprevention of breast cancer. However, the use of tamoxifen as a chemoprevention agent in healthy women would depend on confirmation of its low toxicity and high safety profile trials.

Acute toxicity

Since its introduction for treatment in 1971, reports of acute toxicity for tamoxifen have been few. In a pilot chemoprevention trial conducted at the Royal Marsden Hospital, Surrey, UK, 2500 healthy women who were at high risk of developing breast cancer were randomized to receive either tamoxifen 20 mg/day or placebo (Powles *et al.* 1994). The main side-effects of tamoxifen vs placebo were hot flushes (34% vs 24%), especially in premenopausal women, vaginal discharge (16% vs 4%), and menstrual irregularities (14% vs 9%). As a consequence of the low acute symptomatic toxicity, compliance between the two groups was correspondingly high with 77% of women in the tamoxifen group and 82% in the placebo group continuing medication at 5 years.

Beneficial long-term effects

Serum cholesterol

Several studies have demonstrated a decrease in serum cholesterol levels by approximately 15–20% of pretreatment values and a marked improvement in the serum lipid profile of post-menopausal women (Powles *et al.* 1990; Thangaraju *et al.* 1994; Ilanchazhian *et al.* 1995; Morales *et al.* 1996). The reduction in serum cholesterol levels is similar to that seen during the administration of hormone replacement therapy, indicating that tamoxifen may have an oestrogenic effect on cholesterol metabolism in the liver (Bush *et al.* 1988). The favourable changes in lipid profile are maintained throughout the duration of tamoxifen use in postmenopausal women and could be the basis for the observed reduction in incidence of myocardial infarctions (Love *et al.* 1994; McDonald *et al.* 1995; Costantino *et al.* 1997).

Coagulation factors

A significant reduction in plasma fibrinogen, antithrombin III, and cross-linked fibrinogen degradation products was seen in the Royal Marsden Hospital's pilot chemoprevention study comparing tamoxifen and placebo (Jones *et al.* 1992) and a reduction in plasma fibrinogen (Powles *et al.* 1994). However, the relevance of such a reduction is unknown as a decrease in thromboembolic events has not been witnessed. In fact, contrary to this, some groups have reported an increase in thromboembolic events (Fisher *et al.* 1989*a*; McDonald *et al.* 1995). Only further analysis of the incidence of thromboembolic events in healthy women within ongoing randomized placebo controlled trials using tamoxifen can address this issue.

Bone mineral density

Three randomized placebo controlled trials have demonstrated an encouraging increase in bone mineral density in postmenopausal women (Love *et al.* 1992; Kristensen *et al.* 1994; Powles *et al.* 1996). The increase in spinal bone density and the stabilization of the cortical bone mass in the femoral neck that is seen during treatment with tamoxifen is similar to that seen during hormone replacement therapy, indicating an oestrogenic effect of tamoxifen on bone in postmenopausal women. However, in premenopausal women the contrary is true, with a transient, but significant, reduction in bone mineral density of the lumbar spine and hip being seen in the first two years of medication (Powles *et al.* 1996). This transient effect may have important clinical implications for the future and long-term follow-up of these patients is required.

Long-term risks

Gynaecological effects

Tamoxifen has an oestrogenic effect on the endometrium in postmenopausal women, causing thickening with an increased risk of atypical hyperplasia, which may be associated with an increased risk of endometrial carcinoma. Three large randomized studies have demonstrated a significantly increased risk of endometrial cancer, using tamoxifen 20 mg/day, 30 mg/day, or 40 mg/day, respectively (Fisher *et al.* 1994; Andersson *et al.* 1991; Fornander *et al.* 1989). Other studies have failed to show a significant increase in endometrial carcinoma (Boccardo *et al.* 1992; Ribeiro and Swindell 1992; Stewart 1992).

Women who have developed endometrial carcinoma while on tamoxifen have the diagnosis made at an earlier stage and the carcinomas are of low malignancy grade, suggesting that the prognosis is similar to, or possibly better than, the average for endometrial carcinoma. Nevertheless, there is sufficient evidence from randomized trial data to warrant further exploration of the relationship between tamoxifen use and risk of endometrial carcinoma, and if such a relationship exists, whether it is a causal one. Such questions should be answered adequately before tamoxifen is administered to healthy women outside the context of a clinical trial.

Other potential carcinogenic effects

The genotoxic activity of tamoxifen depends on activation by cytochrome p450 drug-metabolizing enzymes which form reactive intermediates that bind covalently to DNA to create adducts (Han and Liehr 1992) and subsequent DNA damage (White *et al.* 1992; 1995; Pathak and Bodell 1994; Phillips *et al.* 1994). Experimentally, tamoxifen has been shown to cause hepatocellular carcinoma only in certain strains of rat (Robinson *et al.* 1991; Hard *et al.* 1993). However, these experimental data do not allow any prediction of carcinogenic risk to humans. At the present time, tamoxifen should be considered potentially carcinogenic in humans and careful long-term surveillance of clinical trials is required to evaluate the human risk (Powles and Hickish 1995). Adjuvant trials from Scandinavia suggest a possible increase in gastrointestinal tumours in women on 40 mg tamoxifen per day (Rutqvist *et al.* 1995) but no other clinical trials have indicated that tamoxifen acts as a carcinogen outside the female genital tract.

Rare side-effects

Tamoxifen has been reported to cause ocular complications including cataracts, retinopathy and corneal deposits although it is uncommon in the current setting of long-term, low-dose use (Palvidis *et al.* 1992; Nayfield and Gorling 1996; Tang *et al.* 1997). In the majority of cases, the visual disturbance is reversible after cessation of treatment.

In summary, tamoxifen is a well-tolerated drug with high compliance and few acute side-effects. It may have clinically beneficial effects by reducing cholesterol levels and increasing bone mineral density in postmenopausal women. In contrast, clinical evidence indicates a probable increase in thromboembolic events together with an increase in the risk of endometrial carcinoma.

It would appear that the potential benefits of using tamoxifen in women at high risk of developing breast cancer probably outweigh the possible risks.

Royal Marsden NHS Trust pilot study

Before large national trials could be initiated to examine tamoxifen as a chemoprevention agent in breast cancer, a feasibility pilot trial needed to be undertaken. This was commenced in

1986 at The Royal Marsden Hospital, Sutton, UK to evaluate the acceptability, compliance, toxicity, and safety of tamoxifen use in healthy women (Powles *et al.* 1994). Women were randomized to receive tamoxifen 20 mg/day or placebo for up to eight years. This study confirmed that acute symptomatic toxicity was low in the tamoxifen-treated group, with an associated high level of compliance, and that clinical trials of tamoxifen in healthy women were possible.

Multinational trials

Following the completion of the pilot trial at The Royal Marsden Hospital, several large multicentre trials were commenced to evaluate the risks and benefits of tamoxifen in healthy women. The entry criteria for the Italian trial were confined to healthy women aged 50–60 years who had previously undergone hysterectomy but who had no risk factors of developing breast cancer. This trial has accrued approximately 4000 women. In the UK, over 2500 women with approximately a threefold risk of breast cancer because of a family history have been enrolled as part of a multicentre trial involving centres in UK, Europe, and Australia. In addition, the National Surgical Adjuvant Breast and Bowel Project group (NSABP) in the US has been conducting a multicentre trial and has recently released its results after premature closure.

NSABP breast cancer prevention trial

The National Surgical Adjuvant Breast and Bowel Project (NSABP) commenced its breast cancer prevention trial (BCPT) in April 1992. The investigators have recently issued a press release (6 April 1998) with its results, 14 months earlier than expected. This trial involved more than 300 different centres across the US and Canada and recruited 13 388 women within a randomized controlled study comparing tamoxifen 20 mg/day to placebo.

Women aged over 60 qualified on the basis of age alone (as the expected incidence of developing breast cancer is about 17 per 1000 women in five years). Women aged between 35 and 59 required a risk of developing breast cancer equivalent to that of a women aged 60 or over to qualify; the risk was calculated using the multivariate risk Gail model (Gail *et al.* 1989). The risk factors used to assess potential participants were age, number of first-degree relatives diagnosed with breast cancer, age at menarche, parity, age at first delivery, number of times the participant had breast lumps biopsied, particularly if shown to be atypical hyperplasia, and presence of lobular carcinoma *in situ* (Redmond and Costantino 1996). Ethnic minority groups such as African American, Asian American, and Hispanic were poorly represented, making up approximately 3% of participants. Median follow-up was approximately four years with 57% of women receiving tamoxifen or placebo for four or more years.

The results of the trial show that 85 women in the tamoxifen group developed breast cancer compared with 154 in the control group, with three women dying from breast cancer in the tamoxifen group compared with five in the control group. There was a decreased incidence of ductal carcinoma *in situ* (DCIS) in the tamoxifen group with the diagnosis being made in 31 women compared with 59 in the control group. Additional encouraging results include a decrease in the incidence of bone fractures, with 47 women having fractures in the tamoxifen group compared with 71 in the control group. The incidence of myocardial infarctions was not altered between the two cohorts.

However, there were significant adverse effects seen in the tamoxifen group. The incidence of endometrial cancer was increased (33 compared with 14 in the control group), as was the incidence of pulmonary emboli (17 compared with six in the control group) and deep vein thrombosis (30 compared with 19 in the control group).

Patients in the control group of the NSABP trial have already been informed that they are taking a placebo and, as a result, several questions remain unanswered. The follow-up period is insufficient to estimate the long-term risks of tamoxifen treatment. In addition, this study has not, so far, determined whether tamoxifen is equally effective in preventing breast cancer in all risk groups. There is some evidence that those women carrying germ-line *BRCA* mutations in high-risk families are more likely to develop hormone-independent tumours which would probably be resistant to the preventive effects of tamoxifen (Karp *et al.* 1997; Verhoog *et al.* 1998).

Nonetheless, the results from this NSABP trial appear encouraging, although at this time it cannot be concluded that the evidence is sufficient for widespread use of tamoxifen in healthy women. The reduction in incidence of breast cancer in the trial (45%) does not necessarily result in a reduction in mortality, the primary aim of chemoprevention of breast cancer. Breast cancer tumours in women taking tamoxifen may have a worse prognosis due to the selection of tamoxifen-resistant tumours and there is a possibility that only well-differentiated cancers are prevented by tamoxifen.

Conclusion

It is most important to examine closely the side-effects of any drug that could potentially be used as a chemoprevention agent in a clinical trial. Stringent safety monitoring is required if large numbers of healthy women are to be treated for a potential benefit in relatively few.

Tamoxifen has been used to treat women with breast cancer for more than 25 years with relatively few side-effects. It has been shown to decrease recurrent and contralateral breast cancer in both premenopausal and postmenopausal women (Early Breast Cancer Trialists' Collaborative Group 1992; Fisher *et al.* 1994). It increases bone mineral density and decreases the risk of ischaemic heart disease in postmenopausal women. In premenopausal women, there is possibly a detrimental effect on bone mineral density while postmenopausal women probably have an increased risk of thromboembolic events and endometrial cancer. These problems may limit its use as a chemoprevention agent in healthy women and encourage clinical research into other similar agents which may have a more favourable spectrum of activity.

Chemoprevention—a personal perspective

Geraldine

In 1981 I found a breast lump. My mind whirled. I was 41 years old. My youngest child was only two years old. People like me don't get breast cancer, or do they? My GP was very sympathetic and arranged an early appointment to see the consultant at the breast clinic. The breast was duly examined and it was decided to aspirate the lump. I was reassured it would probably be 'all right'. Even with all the reassurance it was difficult not to feel anxious. Surgery followed quickly and the offending lump was removed. Still the anxiety continued until the result came through and thankfully the result of the biopsy showed that it was benign. I was very fortunate in having sympathetic medical staff and a quick follow-through to surgery. As a result of this experience I became much more aware of breast cancer and the consequences. I examined my breasts routinely and had regular checkups at the breast clinic.

Then in 1982 my mother, aged 67, died of breast cancer. She had suffered from a viral encephalitis some 30 years before and as a result did not know any of her family or friends. She received the best of medical attention at the time, but there was nothing that could be done for her. She was in the early stages of her fifth pregnancy and my youngest brother was duly born some months later, a healthy son. She lived the remaining years in the care of loving nuns in a nursing home in Ireland. We grew up in England with holidays in Ireland. It was very emotionally difficult to visit her, she was still the mother we remembered but she didn't know us as her children, so the visits became less frequent. My mother developed a breast lump which was malignant and as a result she had a mastectomy. Some few months later she was dead. It was a sad time but perhaps not as difficult as it might have been if she had been living with us and we had known her better. The loss was greater at the onset of her first illness.

My mother's death made me think more about breast cancer—the whys and the wherefores. Her life in the nursing home would have been relatively stress free but she was a smoker and I think she started smoking before her marriage. I wasn't aware of any previous family history, but it may be that this was something families did not talk about. Some years later my maternal aunt had a mastectomy but she lived a further 12 years, eventually dying of heart failure with no mention of any further cancer.

In 1990 my younger sister, aged 43, found a breast lump. I think we all thought it would be benign just as mine had been but a biopsy confirmed it was malignant. My sister had a local excision and dissection of lymph nodes as well as removal of her ovaries, radiotherapy, and chemotherapy. So much happened in a short period of time. It was impossible to absorb the enormity of it all but we still felt the cancer would be cured as so much progress was being made in the treatment of cancer. We had great hope at the time but our hopes were brutally dashed when secondaries were diagnosed in the lower spine and pelvis. Just two months after her diagnosis she was barely able to walk and very soon after not able to walk at all. My sister was married but had no children. Her husband dealt with her doctors so I did not have any direct contact with them but I know that they were given all the help and advice they sought. My sister spent the last seven weeks of her life in hospital. This was a time none of us would wish to repeat. She suffered from nausea and severe pain which were eventually brought under control. We all experienced frustration, highs, lows, remorse, memories, thoughts shared, some not shared, so many experiences during that time, so much emotion and most of all so much prayer.

Two years later at one of my regular checkups I was asked if I would be interested in joining a chemoprevention trial involving the drug tamoxifen. I knew very little about tamoxifen, just that it was a drug given to women who had breast cancer. I thought that I should at least find out more so I was introduced to the coordinator of the trial and given more information on the trial and tamoxifen. I was told that it was an established therapy in already diagnosed cases of breast cancer and that the purpose of the trial was to see if it could be used to prevent the disease in high-risk, healthy women. I fulfilled the criteria for the trial. I was in the right age bracket, had a family history of breast cancer, and was not considering any more children. I took the information home with me to read in my own time and discuss with my husband. The information explained the action of the drug, the possible side-effects, and the format of the trial. If I accepted I would take the tablet for five years and have regular scans, mammograms, and blood tests.

We discussed all of the pros and cons at great length. I spoke to many friends, discussing what they would do in a similar situation but at the end of the day the decision had to be mine alone. One reassuring fact was that throughout the trial and the 10 year follow-up I was being very carefully monitored and anything abnormal would be picked up. Looking back I think it might have been helpful to have spoken to some of the other women on the trial. I would have also appreciated some further input from the doctors at the time. In the end I came to the conclusion that the advantages outweighed the disadvantages and eventually I decided to give it a go. My decision was made in the hope that no woman would have to go through what my sister suffered. My decision was also made for my daughter and the next generation so they would not have the fears we have today. This was based on a deep hope that this trial might find the answer to this dreadful disease.

So, I started the Tamoplac trial. In the early stages I seemed to have more headaches than usual, but as a person who suffers from headaches I did not worry unduly and within a short time they ceased to be a problem. Soon after I was suffering from very uncomfortable vaginal dryness, followed by hot flushes and night sweats. Having these menopausal symptoms made me suspect I was taking the tamoxifen and not the placebo. As a result of the discomfort associated with these side-effects I felt I had two options: one to discontinue the trial, the other to take up the offer of HRT made to me when I started the study. My instinct was to continue with the trial but I knew of the association between HRT and breast cancer and that worried me. At my next appointment I discussed these worries with my doctor. It was explained that HRT would not lead to a significantly increased risk if taken for a short five-year course, and regular monitoring would detect any problems. The initial low-dose HRT hardly made any difference but once the dose was increased things greatly improved and life got back to a regular pattern again.

During all this time I had every support from the trial coordinator; she was and still is always at the other end of the telephone if I need any advice. At every appointment I saw a new doctor which did not assist continuity or the development of a relationship with a particular doctor. Newsletters come at regular intervals and there was one get-together of participants in 1993. I found the meeting very informative and helpful. I really enjoyed meeting some of the other women involved.

The trial was originally for five years, but coming up to the fifth year there was no discussion as to whether it would be continued or not. Of my own volition and after five and a half years I decided to stop taking HRT. Although I was reassured it was

11
Surgical treatment options

A. Skene

Introduction

Contemporary diagnosis of breast cancer is based on clinical, imaging, and cytological assessments (triple assessment) of selected breast abnormalities. This initial evaluation in the majority of specialized breast clinics is led by surgeons; it is, however, their role as a surgical oncologist rather than a surgical operator that brings most influence to the surgical decision-making process.

After initial triple assessment, over 90% of women with breast cancer can have a preoperative diagnosis. However, these patients are inevitably burdened by having to absorb the implications of a preoperative diagnosis, concurrent with discussing treatment options.

Although the management of breast cancer is best formulated within the context of a multidisciplinary team, it is frequently the surgeon who initially conveys this information to the patient, since surgery remains the main treatment modality in the local control of breast cancer. The timing and extent of surgery are, however, influenced not only by the stage of disease at presentation but also by the required aims and choices of treatment offered.

Surgery for breast cancer has survived the legacy of the time when increasingly radical mastectomy operations were advocated. These treatments were based on the false hypothesis of radial spread from local disease to regional lymphatics and from there to systemic sites. Currently, even with a far greater understanding of tumour biology, a modified mastectomy remains a very important contemporary operative option in the local control of breast cancer. In many specialist units when mastectomy is recommended this can be offered in conjunction with immediate breast reconstruction. Although reconstruction may partially compensate for the ablative component of such treatment, it adds to the complexity with additional treatment choices.

When considering a patient for breast-conserving surgery, traditional selection criteria have been based on didactic factors heavily biased towards the tumour itself. These criteria are commonly listed in both undergraduate and postgraduate textbooks. However, these factors are relative indicators and should not be seen as prescriptive. The influence of a women's preference in determining her treatment is equally pertinent. The clinician's role is to advise what is oncologically acceptable and to discuss the long-term implications, benefits, and risks. The main price of adoption of conservative surgery against these criteria is often at the expense of long-term local recurrence rates and cosmesis.

Summary of the present situation in breast cancer surgical treatment options

The initial decision to be taken by the majority of patients with a new breast cancer is in the offer of surgery. Biological and not chronological age should be the determinant of the use of this treatment modality. The main surgical option open to many women with operable breast cancer is whether to have conservative surgery or a mastectomy. A fully informed patient may, however, elect to have a mastectomy even if conservative surgery could offer a good chance of local disease control. This decision should not be based on the mistaken belief that the more radical operation proffers a significantly greater chance of long-term survival. The psychological morbidity following traditional breast cancer surgery is well documented. When these treatments invariably involved mastectomy, it was tempting to relate these psychological effects to the loss of body image with such ablative treatments. Subsequent studies have shown a similar degree of morbidity following conservative surgery, concluding that psychological morbidity is related to the events of diagnosis and therapy rather than the external manifestation of one particular operation. Breast reconstruction can reduce the morbidity following mastectomy and should routinely be discussed with all patients when this surgical treatment is offered. The majority of techniques for breast reconstruction utilize either tissue expansion or myocutaneous flap transfer. Each of these methods has benefits and risks which need to be discussed, adding further complexity to the decision-making process.

When counselling a patient about surgical treatment options, tumour size is still a significant factor. Most surgeons would advise a women with a tumour clinically greater than 4–5 cm in diameter to consider a mastectomy in preference to breast-conserving surgery. The main reason being that removal of a 2-cm margin of normal breast tissue surrounding these tumours would produce an unacceptable cosmetic result if conservative surgery were attempted. Indeed, within a small breast such a resection may constitute a near total mastectomy. Women with small breasts or those with large tumours are less likely to benefit from breast-preserving surgery and should be preoperatively counselled regarding the potential progressive cosmetic deformity. Ultimately, the acceptability of a cosmetic result is the subjective assessment of the women herself.

Women with large-volume breasts are cosmetically more able to tolerate surgical resections required for relatively large tumours. The field and dosimetry planning for subsequent radiotherapy is, however, rendered more difficult. Problems related to radiation tolerance of a fatty breast and the attainment of a uniform dose can result in increased fibrosis and subsequent impaired cosmetic outcome. It is often easier for women with small breasts to relate to the deformity of conservative surgery than for women with large breasts to relate to the potential risks of radiotherapy.

Tumour location remains an important factor in consideration of the type of surgery recommended. Peripheral tumours can often, with appropriately placed incisions, produce good cosmetic results with equal disease control, and can be offered as an alternative to mastectomy. Cancers which require resection of the nipple areolar complex are usually best treated with mastectomy. Central quadrantectomy including the nipple areolar complex can, however, be offered in selected patients, particularly those with large breasts. Patients with multifocal tumours or those with diffuse disease can be offered multiple or generous resections, but the breast is frequently left unacceptably deformed and mastectomy is more usually recommended.

Patients who make a preference to have conservative breast surgery are invariably recommended to have postoperative radiotherapy to reduce the incidence of local recurrence. To be eligible for this approach patients must be able to tolerate radiotherapy treatment positions and be able to complete the course.

Lymph node examination after axillary dissection allows for accurate staging of disease. There is continuing debate as to whether the regional lymph nodes should be sampled or radically excised in patients with breast cancer. It is clear that the more radical the axillary clearance, the more accurate the staging. A full clearance provides precise assessment, reduces the risk of axillary recurrence, and allows the axilla to be excluded from adjuvant radiotherapy fields. Importantly, the histological information obtained from all the nodes in conjunction with that derived from the tumour itself is used to plan the most appropriate adjuvant treatment. The potential complications of seroma, neuralgia from the intercostobrachial nerve, shoulder stiffness, lymphoedema, and inflammatory episodes are balanced with these oncological gains. On the horizon are several methods of preoperatively staging the axilla, with current interest placed in sentinal node biopsy. None of these methods has to date been shown to provide as accurate information as radical axillary dissection.

The timing of surgery can be important in relation to the order of treatment modalities and even to the menstrual cycle. Patients presenting with large (T3) tumours, in whom mastectomy would be the only reasonable operative treatment, may be offered consideration for primary medical therapy where the surgical component is deferred, the rationale of such therapy being both early systemic protection and downstaging of the primary tumour. Significant downstaging may shrink the tumour to a point where conservative surgery can be offered. A small proportion of patients with primary chemotherapy downstage at the end of the course to the point where there is no evaluable disease. In these patients surgery can be avoided altogether, and consolidation radiotherapy offered to give additional protection to the breast.

One study suggested that survival following surgery was improved in premenopausal women if the operation was delayed to coincide with the luteal phase of the menstrual cycle. These results have not been consistently reproduced and most centres offer surgery at the first available opportunity.

Additional surgical options may be offered as part of adjuvant treatment and for advanced disease. Premenopausal women with oestrogen-receptor-positive tumours may be recommended to have endocrine manipulations. The aim of such treatment is to render the patient menopausal. This can be achieved by a variety of treatment modalities including LH-RH analogue injections, pelvic radiotherapy, and surgical oophorectomy. Surgery offers a permanent treatment and, particularly with laparoscopic techniques, can be performed with minimal morbidity.

Some salvage surgical procedures may be offered in advanced disease, for example, a chest wall resection for a locally advanced tumour deposit. The aim is to palliate uncontrolled local or recurrent disease rather than to increase life expectancy. The benefit-risk balance of salvage surgical procedures is suited to discussion at multidisciplinary meetings but is a difficult concept for patients to assess, since they may have little insight into the problem of uncontrolled locoregional disease.

The point in time and stage at which a women presents herself with breast cancer shows great variation. Once she has presented, her expectation is of rapid diagnosis and this can be realized in the majority of cases by triple assessment in the specialist breast clinic. The desire and delivery of a prompt diagnosis reduces the time available for coming to terms with the implications of the diagnosis, including treatment options. This is most graphically demonstrated in a one-stop diagnostic breast clinic, which in itself can be a major cause of morbidity. Women must have time to consider the treatment options.

Once breast cancer is diagnosed, treatment decisions nevertheless have to be taken at a time when a woman may feel vulnerable. The specialist and team have an obligation to provide information in a way that can be interpreted. Breast care nurses have an established role in the management of breast cancer. They assist patients with the implications of the diagnosis and with treatment options. They offer counselling and emotional support and provide a variety of clinical and organizational roles. There is good evidence that the psychological distress in patients with serious illness is less when they have received adequate information.

The clinical team must facilitate free two-way communication and discuss realistic treatment choices. An important consideration is how the information relates to the patient in her own case. This requires individual knowledge and background details. These issues may be difficult to discuss within the time constraints of a clinical setting where communication often has a lower priority than medical treatment. Most women want to take part in treatments that fit with their moral values, their work and social circumstances, and their responsibilities towards themselves and their families.

Invariably, prior to a detailed discussion on surgical treatment options there is a review of the general oncological status. Nearly all patients wish to know if the results show a breast cancer (96%), the potential for cure (91%), and the side-effects of treatment (94%). While the majority of patients (79%) wish to know everything, not all do and their wishes must be respected. The woman's desire for information does not tell the oncologist how to break bad news. Theory can clarify choices but cannot offer a solution to the question of how these choices should be made. There is great variance in the wish to participate in treatment options. The first choice is whether the woman wishes to be actively involved in the treatment process.

Kate and Richard—personal views

Kate's experience

Four years ago at the age of 32 I was diagnosed with breast cancer. In reviewing the process of treatment decisions, I felt that overall my experience had been a positive one as I will outline below.

It must, however, be said that the experience did not start out so positively! The first surgeon I saw gave a very negative first impression. He seemed pompous and uncaring in his attitude. He made me feel stupid that I was concerned about the lump I found in my breast. At the interview I plucked up the courage to ask him if he felt there was any possibility of there being something seriously wrong. He dismissed the whole idea. At the time, I was not ever offered an ultrasound or mammogram, and he very reluctantly agreed to put me on the list to have the lump removed. I felt I was denied the possibility of screening because I was young and young people do not get breast cancer! At least that was what I was told.

Just before the lump was removed, a new consultant came to the hospital where I was being treated. His whole approach was very different. He had recently come from a well-known Cancer Centre, and I was immediately very glad to be under his care. I met him on the morning I was to have the lump removed. When it had been removed and I was told the diagnosis, my new breast surgeon, proposed a quadrantectomy and axillary clearance. He *took time* to explain the reasons why and then arranged an ultrasound and mammogram. He *spent time*, explaining my situation and possible outcomes after the initial surgery, and the various treatment options available. He also *spent time* listening to my questions, of which there were a multitude, and took the time to answer them. My questions ranged from wanting to know the prognosis, my risks of recurrence and mortality expectations, to how long I should stay in hospital and could the children visit. I felt that the only reason I knew what and how to ask was because I have a medical training myself.

My new surgeon never gave me the impression that he felt my questions were invalid or unimportant. His relaxed but professional attitude filled me with confidence. I never felt that he was too rushed to talk, that he was trying to fob me off with any old answer, or that he was being anything but 100% honest.

When the results of the surgery were known I had various options open to me. I had an idea of what they were because they had been planted like seeds in my mind along the way. Just prior to going to the theatre for surgery, I was informed I would need a course of radiotherapy and that the doctors might want to 'play around' with my hormones. At the time I only had a vague notion as to what this might mean.

After the surgery, the course of radiotherapy was arranged and again I found those dealing with me to be very kind and willing to discuss my questions and concerns.

As I recall, the options open to me were:

(1) to take part in a CRC trial comparing zoladex and tamoxifen;
(2) monthly zoladex injections or ovarian oblation;
(3) to take tamoxifen for two, but probably five, years;
(4) bilateral mastectomy in view of 'mirror imaging' in the particular type of breast cancer that I had.

It became obvious after further lengthy discussions that my surgeon's preference was that I should take tamoxifen and have my ovaries removed. I started the tamoxifen immediately. I knew from reading the recent research at the time that it seemed the oophorectomy was the best thing to do, but found the whole concept of artificial menopause, more surgery, and coping with three small children extremely difficult to come to terms with.

My surgeon did not make the decision for me but gave me time to think it all through. At the time I was also helped by my GP and a friend who had expertise in the whole area. The latter encouraged me at each point of the decision-making process. At the same time, I was seeing a privately arranged counsellor whom I found very helpful. His main advice was to do all in my power to prolong my life or lessen the risks because of my children who were aged four, two, and one year old at the time. These decisions were not taken lightly and caused great anguish. However, six months after the initial surgery I felt ready to consent to an oophorectomy.

I am sure that being involved in the decision-making process has helped me make such a good recovery. I am very grateful to those who cared and still care for me.

Richard's experience

A view from the other side (the husband)!
My wife did not reveal the level of her concern about the lump for a long time, and barely admitted to me that it could be cancer. This being the case, I was actually away when she received the diagnosis and I was not able to be present to support her at that time. Receiving the news over the 'phone was devastating and a variety of emotions swept through me, and us as we reunited.

I too want to acknowledge and praise the extremely competent level of care and help she received during the decision-making process. We are where we are today because of this expertise and because of our faith in God which sustained us throughout, even though only just at times!

If I felt there were any areas of lack it was in terms of emotional support and counselling for us as a couple. There was a breast care counsellor offered but the emphasis was placed on us calling for help and taking the initiative. It is often difficult to ask questions that you do not know are going to exist. My wife has a medical training and that helped. I do not believe she would have made such an informed choice if she had not had that background or the personal support of her friend, whose expertise is in this area.

In addition, I do not feel that the full extent of the effects of the oophorectomy were fully explained. Since that time she has experienced insufferable hot flushes, vulnerability to minor illnesses, and also endured a period of depression. Nothing prepared us for those, and no-one spoke to us about the possible effects on our relationship, emotionally and physically.

12

Early breast cancer—medical treatment options

I.E. Smith

Background

The most significant advance in breast cancer management during the last quarter century has come from the realization that this is a systemic disease from the outset in the majority of patients. In other words most patients, when they first present with a malignant lump to the breast, already have microscopic metastases which have spread, principally through the blood, to other parts of the body. This means that systemic medical treatments are usually required in addition to (or as adjuvant to) local treatment to the breast itself.

Clinical trials involving tens of thousands of patients with early breast cancer have reinforced these points, and two major conclusions have emerged from these trials. First, the intensity of local treatment (conservative surgery, mastectomy, axillary resection, postoperative radiotherapy, etc.) may influence local control rates, but does not influence survival. Second, adjuvant medical treatments do significantly influence survival. In absolute terms the influence is usually small, of the order of 5–10% absolute difference. Given the high incidence of breast cancer, particularly in Western nations, these differences are important and translate into thousands of lives saved per year.

Ovarian ablation was one of the earliest forms of adjuvant therapy to be used in early breast cancer and now dates back almost 50 years. This has been shown to achieve a significant survival benefit in premenopausal patients but at the cost of early menopause with associated symptoms and, of course, permanent infertility.

The antioestrogen tamoxifen also has an established role as adjuvant therapy and achieves a significant survival benefit.

The benefit appears greatest in patients whose tumour is oestrogen receptor rich. In addition, older women appear to achieve a greater benefit than younger women, although this at least to some extent relates to oestrogen receptor status. Current evidence suggests that there is no benefit for adjuvant tamoxifen in women under the age of 50 whose tumours are oestrogen receptor negative, and evidence is emerging that tamoxifen may be of little or no benefit in any woman whose tumour is oestrogen receptor negative.

The duration of adjuvant tamoxifen treatment remains a matter of some debate. Current trials indicates a slight survival advantage for five years of treatment versus two years. The issue of tamoxifen prolonged for more than five years is controversial. At least two trials have failed to show further benefit and furthermore there is the hint, no more, that treatment prolonged beyond five years may slightly decrease survival. There is some scientific basis to explain this apparent paradox. In experimental tumour models, tamoxifen can be demonstrated to become agonistic rather than antagonistic with prolonged use.

Adjuvant chemotherapy has also been shown to be of significant survival benefit in all subgroups of women so far assessed under the age of 70. The benefit, however, decreases with age and is greatest in younger women, particularly under the age of 50. This is important because chemotherapy, unlike tamoxifen, has significant side-effects. Some of these, and in particular bone marrow suppression, are greater in older women. Important issues remain in determining the optimum form of chemotherapy. CMF (Cyclophosphamide, Methotrexate, 5-FU) is accepted as the 'gold standard'. The weight of current data suggests that anthracycline-containing chemotherapy has a marginal advantage over CMF. Six courses of chemotherapy are as effective as 12 and there are some data to suggest that three or four courses may be as good as six. At least one trial has shown that a single course of peroperative chemotherapy is less effective than several courses.

High-dose chemotherapy with peripheral blood stem cell rescue currently has a high profile. It is sometimes advocated for high-risk patients, e.g. with multiple node positive disease, particularly in the USA. Enthusiasm for this stems from non-randomized pilot studies which were compared with historical controls. Currently, several large randomized trials of high-dose chemotherapy are underway, both in the US and Europe. At present no data are available; however, the data emerging from a large US trial suggests that the benefit, if any, is unlikely to be dramatic. For the time being, therefore, this approach should be considered entirely experimental and is not to be recommended outside the context of a trial.

There is a weight of evidence to suggest that combined chemotherapy and tamoxifen offers the maximum survival benefit for many patients and this is increasingly becoming standard practice. Exceptions to this are:

(1) women under 50 with oestrogen receptor negative tumours who are best treated with chemotherapy alone;

(2) older women, particularly in their 60s and 70s with oestrogen receptor positive tumours, who are often best treated with tamoxifen alone and who would have little further to gain from the addition of chemotherapy.

There is no hard dividing line here, however, and a value judgement on the addition of chemotherapy often has to be made by each individual patient (see below).

Preoperative medical therapy (sometimes referred to as neoadjuvant or primary therapy) is the most recent development in the medical treatment of early breast cancer. Here the roles are reversed and medical treatment is given before rather than after surgery. The origins of this approach lie within locally advanced breast cancer, where good tumour regressions were consistently achieved with chemotherapy or tamoxifen. Preoperative medical treatment offers the advantage that the tumour can be used as an *in vivo* measure of responsiveness of medical treatment, rather than adjuvant therapy which is given 'blind'. If the primary regresses on treatment then the reasonable hypothesis can be made that putitive micrometastases are also responding to therapy. In addition, preoperative treatment can be used to downstage primary cancers, particularly where mastectomy would be the initial surgical option, in the hopes that conservative surgery can subsequently be achieved.

Preoperative chemotherapy has been widely studied and achieves clinical response rates of around 70–90% depending on the intensity of treatment. Complete clinical remissions occur in 20–50% of patients, but histologically proven, pathological, complete remissions are less common and can be achieved in around 10–20%. Randomized trials have confirmed that preoperative chemotherapy reduces the need for mastectomy. The largest preoperative chemotherapy trial so far published (NSABP-18) has so far shown that survival is the same whether treatment is given pre- or postoperatively. The need for mastectomy in this trial was, however, significantly reduced. Tamoxifen instead of surgery has been assessed in several trials over the last 10–15 years, particularly in elderly patients. Tamoxifen alone has, however, been consistently shown to result in a high local relapse rate and this treatment is not recommended except in the very elderly and frail. Tamoxifen before surgery has been less extensively investigated, but trials are now underway to assess the value of this approach, particularly in older patients with oestrogen receptor positive tumours in which chemotherapy would be considered inappropriate.

Shared decision-making with patients

Adjuvant tamoxifen

Decision-making on the value of adjuvant tamoxifen is usually relatively straightforward. The survival benefit is clear cut and side-effects are usually fairly minimal, particularly in older women. The media have given an inappropriately high profile to the increased risk of uterine cancer, deep venous thrombosis, and pulmonary embolism. These issues need to be raised with patients but my own argument is based firmly on the established fact that survival benefit clearly outweighs these risks. The risk of uterine cancer remains very low and even when it occurs is usually curable. The key point to be emphasized is that unexplained, postmenopausal bleeding needs investigating. The whole of the data on tamoxifen trials shows two things clearly: first, survival from breast cancer death is improved; and second, there is no evidence of an increased risk of death from other causes.

The main problem in decision-making with tamoxifen usually concerns younger, premenopausal women who can sometimes experience unpleasant side-effects including bleeding, hot flushes, and weight gain. It is important to clarify the cause of hot flushes;

these can sometimes be caused by concurrent chemotherapy-induced amenorrhea and can be wrongly attributed to tamoxifen. If tamoxifen is clearly implicated, then this becomes a value judgement for the individual patient: do these chronic side-effects justify the small increase in survival benefit? In this respect it becomes very important to establish the oestrogen receptor status in such women. If the tumour is oestrogen receptor negative, this is a strong indication to stop treatment.

Adjuvant chemotherapy

In contrast to tamoxifen, adjuvant chemotherapy can provide a real dilemma for many patients; despite an established survival benefit, side-effects can be unpleasant. The problem is compounded by the fact that chemotherapy has a 'bad name'. Many women have heard of numerous unpleasant experiences caused by chemotherapy and are not surprisingly very anxious about this treatment. In my experience, the approach here is to discuss carefully the nature of the side-effects and how these can be minimized. In addition, the value of discussions with an experienced nurse specialist on this topic can't be overemphasized.

The 5HT3 antagonists, granisetron and ondansetron, have greatly helped to reduce nausea and vomiting, and for many patients this problem is a minimal one. If an anthracycline such as adriamycin is used, scalp cooling can sometimes prevent socially unacceptable alopecia, or at least shorten its duration. For many patients the main problem with chemotherapy is fatigue. If this is discussed carefully beforehand and advice given to take plenty of rest for two or three days after treatment, then the impact of this can be reduced.

Nowadays, several different adjuvant chemotherapy options are available, with differing side-effects. CMF is still the most commonly used schedule, particularly in the UK, and usually avoids alopecia. It is important to note, however, that the best effects are achieved with gold standard or so-called 'classical' CMF, and yet this schedule is in fact quite toxic. My own experience is that an anthracycline-containing schedule is often better tolerated and means less clinic visits, providing the short-term risk of alopecia is accepted. The MM schedule of mitozantrone and methotrexate, although not as widely tested as adriamycin against conventional schedules, can also be used with only a small risk of alopecia.

Duration of treatment is an important issue. Nowadays there is no basis for going on beyond six courses and it may be that three or four courses are as effective. Again, in my own personal experience I find that patients can accept the prospect of chemotherapy more readily if they aim initially at four courses with the option of a further two provided treatment is going well.

One of the most important papers concerning decision-making in adjuvant chemotherapy was published by Sleven *et al.* (1990). The authors compared the attitudes to chemotherapy of patients with cancer to those of doctors, nurses, and the general public. The most striking finding was that patients were willing to accept strong chemotherapy even if the chances of benefit were extremely small (e.g. a 1% increase in the chance of cure). In contrast, doctors and nurses, for whom the question was merely hypothetical, were much less likely to accept such treatment unless the chances of cure were greater (10–50%).

This important study cautioned against common current practice whereby doctors decide among themselves whether or not it is worth offering adjuvant chemotherapy to patients. Adjuvant chemotherapy initially, is as much like any other medical treatment options in breast cancer medicine where the decision-making process must be shared with the patient. Slevin's results are often assessed with scepticism but my own experience strongly suggests that he is right: the great majority of patients with whom I discuss adjuvant chemotherapy opt for this treatment, although they understand clearly that the additional survival benefits may be fairly marginal.

Adjuvant chemotherapy and infertility

Fortunately this issue affects only a relatively small number of younger patients, but when it arises it presents one of the most difficult treatment decisions. Adjuvant chemotherapy carries a degree of infertility risk for almost all women but the risk is strongly age related. For a woman in her forties, permanent chemotherapy-induced amenorrhea is very likely. This risk diminishes in younger age-groups; it is about 50% around the age of 35 and less than 25% in women 30 and under. The problem is that even a 20% risk of permanent infertility can be of great additional anguish to a young women faced with the anxiety of breast cancer. The issue is compounded by the fact that current techniques of *in vitro* embryo storage carry their own problems: ovum fertilization before storage is required—the process takes several weeks which means delay in starting treatment, oestrogen stimulation is required which could, in theory at least, enhance residual tumour growth, and finally, the success rate of *in vitro* fertilization remains low, at around 20%. There are no easy answers here. The first step is to ensure that the patient has all the facts clearly presented. Social issues also play an important part in the equation. A woman who already has a husband and dependent young family may feel that her priority lies in going for the best chance at a cure even if it carries the risk of no further children; in contrast a young single woman may prefer to undergo harvesting and storage (providing she has the partner for fertilization) or even not have chemotherapy rather than jeopardize her chance of child bearing. Although different chemotherapy options are currently available as described above, so far none has been clearly identified as carrying a significantly reduced risk of infertility.

Adjuvant oophorectomy

Adjuvant oophorectomy seems to me, personally, a rather unattractive option for most patients. It is certainly of survival benefit, but currently there are no data to suggest that this is any more effective than chemotherapy and/or tamoxifen. It carries a certainty of infertility, along with the strong likelihood of acute and usually marked menopausal symptoms. Theoretically it also carries the standard long-term risk of early menopause, although to date there are no data to confirm increased long-term risks of osteoporosis and/or cardiovascular disease. Trials are currently underway to see if oophorectomy carries an additional survival benefit when used in conjunction with chemotherapy. Should these trials prove positive, then this whole issue will need further assessment.

Preoperative chemotherapy

Preoperative chemotherapy represents a more recent dilemma in the decision-making process for a woman with breast cancer. At present, most breast cancer specialists would consider this option only in women with larger cancers for whom mastectomy would otherwise prove likely. It is important to note, however, that trials are also being carried out in patients with small cancers. In discussing the pros and cons of preoperative chemotherapy, the most important issue for the doctor to emphasize, as far as I am concerned, is that this is not an 'either or' option. Preoperative chemotherapy should only be offered to patients in whom chemotherapy would be a very likely adjuvant option. In other words, the decision is not about whether to have chemotherapy or surgery, but more simply, in which order to have the two treatments.

The first and most immediate advantage is that chemotherapy offers the possibility of avoiding mastectomy by downstaging the tumour. It is important to emphasize, however, that this is in no way guaranteed. There are already considerable data confirming that mastectomy can be avoided in some or even the majority of patients in the short term; at present we do not have enough long-term follow-up information to assess whether or not this carries an increased long-term risk of recurrence.

The second and perhaps more important potential benefit is that the tumour can be used as an *in vivo* measure of response which has the potential for predicting long-term benefit. Current results consistently show that non-responders to preoperative chemotherapy have a worse prognosis than responders. This therefore offers the individual non-responding patient the option of either stopping or switching to an alternative chemotherapy schedule. Many of us involved in this field are optimistic that in the future we can use this response in a more sophisticated way to determine individual treatment. Most groups are finding that complete pathological remission following surgical resection carries a significantly improved prognosis but this, of course, is not an immediate predictive test. The aim is to establish biological tumour markers of predictive significance for chemotherapy-including markers of apoptosis, proliferation, cerB-2, and the like. If this can be achieved, then preoperative chemotherapy could become a most important tool for optimizing treatment for the individual patient and this is the goal of current research.

The downside of preoperative chemotherapy in the individual patient mainly concerns the absence of standard prognostic information at the time of treatment. Information on axillary nodal involvement is unavailable, and even histological grading is difficult to assess on needle biopsy, and impossible on cytology. Recent data indicate a significant survival benefit for patients with good prognosis just as much as those with poor prognosis and therefore this issue is less important than it was in terms of deciding treatment. For many women, accurate prognostic information simply serves as an additional cause of anxiety and may be undesirable, but others very much want this information and want to know their outlook in detail, for better or for worse. In those, the potential benefits of preoperative chemotherapy may be outweighed by the 'need to know'.

Preoperative endocrine therapy

My own experience of preoperative endocrine therapy is recent and, so far, limited. I am already struck by the confidence that an early tumour regression on tamoxifen gives to both the patient and doctor when recommending prolonged treatment for five years or more. Whether or not this confidence is justified, and whether preoperative treatment can be used to determine whether one form of endocrine therapy is superior to another in an individual patient, are issues that can only be answered after extensive trials.

Conclusions

The management of early breast cancer is complex and often involves several treatment options. In recent years medical treatments have been shown to achieve a significant survival benefit, but the absolute difference in outcome is small. This means that treatment decisions are often based on value judgements that can only be made if the appropriate information is shared between doctor and patient. The role of the nurse specialist in this decision-making process is also extremely important. It is important to note that in the balance between side-effects and benefit, doctors and nurses frequently underestimate what patients are prepared to go through, even for a small increase in the chance of cure.

Medical treatment options—a personal view

Helen

"I'm sorry to have to tell you that you have some very abnormal cells—very abnormal cells indeed . . . and that very quickly you are going to have to decide whether to have a mastectomy or not." With hindsight, I realize that the registrar who delivered this information as he stood at the foot of the bed on which I was sitting, semi-dressed in my half-open blue gown, probably said a great deal more than this, but these words are all I registered in those initial few moments of diagnosis.

It was of course a shock—I was the fittest of all my 40-something contemporaries. I ran four miles several days a week, I'd never smoked, I had a good, if demanding, job, I had supportive family and friends—I was in charge of my life and facing mortality was not on my agenda. Yet, here I was being told that this body—which I was really rather happy with—was in fact producing something 'highly abnormal' and I had a decision to make about whether I was to have an important part of it amputated.

I struggled to assimilate the implications of what I'd been told—surely whether I had a mastectomy or not was not my 'decision'—after all, I knew nothing about the pros and cons of mastectomy other than a dim recollection that I had read somewhere that just as many women died from breast cancer having had mastectomies as those who had not. I also vaguely remembered hearing a radio programme which had highlighted the plight of women who had suffered swelling in their arms after breast cancer surgery, and that the general drift had been that not much could be done about this.

Very quickly the shock transformed into a surge of unfocused anger, which I concentrated into a sequence of questions directed at the registrar who seemed enormously relieved that I was at least asking sensible questions: would I be able to write and use a computer keyboard (it was my right breast—my job depended on being able to do these things), how would anyone know whether the cancer had spread, how soon would I be having surgery and what were the alternatives to mastectomy? The registrar—still standing—was answering as many of these questions as fast as he could when suddenly, to his visible dismay, my facade of reasonable control collapsed and I burst into tears. At which point I remember him urgently saying to the nurse that she should 'get Jan'.

The arrival of the breast care nurse was the first of a number of critical turning points in my treatment. She took control of the situation. She waved the registrar aside as, through my tears, he tried to tell me something, I think to do with where I could get some more information. She was right of course—much as the registrar had accurately identified that I was the kind of patient who wanted as much information as possible, at that very moment all I needed was to deal with the shocking realization that I had cancer.

From this point onwards, as I slowly began to comprehend what was happening, I remember making it insistently clear that I had to find out more about this disease. That because of the kind of person I was, this would be my strategy for coping and regaining control. So how was I to get to grips with what I needed to know? At this point the registrar suggested a sequence of articles on breast cancer that had been running recently in the *BMJ*. He stressed that they were intended for GPs, the nurse said the illustrations were very strong. I said that I thought I could handle that. Within 48 hours I was in the library of the Royal Society for Medicine making detailed notes, compiling a list of questions, and creating a personal glossary that would have done any first-year medic proud.

What happened after this was basically a collaboration between the breast care nurse and myself which helped me understand, as far as was possible for a lay person, the information I was digesting about breast cancer—both about the physical and psychological aspects. This might sound as if it was highly demanding of the breast care nursing team's time. In fact I don't believe this was the case, not least because I was acutely aware of how busy everyone was. There were a couple of occasions when I specifically made an appointment to see the breast care nurse to discuss what I had read, but more often than not, this was done as part of my routine appointments. I'd also got to know a researcher who was regularly at the outpatient's clinic who was extremely helpful in explaining and clarifying issues—not in terms of the specifics of my own case but in providing an overview of what was happening at the research end. The result of all this was that I felt much more confident about what I wanted to discuss in terms of my own particular condition with the various consultants and registrars (and there were many!) that I encountered during the course of my treatment.

The issue of the mastectomy was resolved when I was examined by the professor who happened to present at his clinic when I attended my next visit. He declared that it would be possible to do a lumpectomy. This news seemed too good to be true. To my chagrin I did not question why only a week earlier there had been mention of a mastectomy, and why it no longer seemed to be on the agenda. In situations where there are options, even highly motivated patients who want collaboration and participation with their medical practitioners are only too happy to accept advice without question, if the option being selected is one the patient wants to hear!

Surgery quickly followed. The nodal dissection revealed no visible spread to the nodes—on the other hand the tumour was 1.5 cm in size and had been classified as Grade 3.

At this point, I became part of the clinic of another consultant. He made it clear that the recommendation was that I should undergo a course of chemotherapy followed by radiotherapy. His manner was polite and avuncular—a little knowledge was a dangerous thing. I was advised to follow the recommendation. But I knew that there was a high proportion of cases where chemotherapy would not necessarily be effective—how could I be sure what the weighting of likely effectiveness was to be in my own case? This was something on which I wanted more information and time to consider the factors involved—I was not going to undergo four to six months of potential misery and further serious disruption to my life unless I was fairly confident that there was benefit to be derived from it. From his manner, I knew that this was not something I could easily discuss with this particular consultant.

I was surprised how much anxiety this situation generated. By now I knew how important it was for me to feel that I was being supervised by someone with whom I could talk freely about the pros and cons of various choices. I had also come to understand that decisions in relation to treatment were not nearly as easy or straightforward as might at first seem. Again, I turned to the breast care nurse and talked over the various pros and cons with her. I read some more articles, asked more questions. Was there another consultant I could speak to who might be more empathetic to the approach I needed?

Eventually I was transferred to the clinic of a young oncologist who, although about to move on to another teaching hospital, patiently and openly explored the various reasons for and against the chemotherapy in terms of the facts as they related to my particular case. The relief that I was again being supervised by someone who was prepared to attune themselves to my need for information and open discussion of the options was tremendous.

I did in fact opt for the chemotherapy—despite understanding its potential limitations in terms of preventing recurrence or spread. I was, however, happy with that decision—it had been taken as part of a genuine collaboration between me and my medical team. I had felt that there had been real options concerning whether or not to undergo the chemotherapy and that I had not been pressurized either way. I am convinced that the process of feeling I had made an informed choice at this point in my treatment was absolutely critical to my ability to cope as well as I did with the five months of chemotherapy that followed.

This has continued as an important element as time has elapsed from the original diagnosis. I feel a part of my consultant's team, where this approach of open collaboration underpins the relationship between the medical team and the the patient. During the past two years, I have been seen not only by my consultant but several of the young registrars who have been assisting at his clinics. They have all been unfailingly open and sensitive to my need for information as a means of coping with breast cancer.

I am sure there are many patients who are very happy not to engage so directly with the dicisions about the options available to them during treatment for a condition such as cancer. All I can say is that in my own case, the knowledge that I was able to rely on a combination of information and collaboration when options had to be assessed was vital in helping me maintain a healthy and realistic approach to my illness. Like any patient who has had cancer, I think from time to time about the possibility of recurrence. For me, if that time comes, knowing that I can rely on an approach based around open, shared decision-making will play a vital role in my ability to cope.

13

Radiotherapy treatment

G. McPhail and T. Habeshaw

Radiotherapy as an adjuvant treatment for early breast cancer

Mastectomy was the treatment of choice for breast cancer until the results of randomized clinical trials published in the 1980s demonstrated no difference in overall survival in women treated by mastectomy or breast-conserving treatment (Veronesi *et al.* 1981; Fisher *et al.* 1985). Fisher *et al.* (1989) subsequently demonstrated that those women who received radiotherapy following breast-conserving surgery had significantly lower local recurrence rates (5% vs 30%). As a result of these clinical trials, women with early breast cancer now typically have a choice of local treatment with either mastectomy or breast-conserving treatment (Street *et al.* 1995), although Bergh (1997) points out that 60–70% of women receiving breast-conserving treatment may be overtreated, because they will not experience disease relapse irrespective of postoperative radiation therapy.

Recognition of the issue of patient choice not only reflects developments in our understanding of breast cancer, but also the marked cultural changes that have occurred in Europe and the US over recent decades, demonstrating increasing concern for individual autonomy and consumer rights (Richards *et al.* 1995). Feldman *et al.* (1997) surmize that breast cancer treatment choices have acquired a quasi-political flavour, owing to the advent of an active patient advocacy movement.

When breast-conserving treatment was first acknowledged as a valid alternative to mastectomy for women with early breast cancer, it was widely assumed that the majority of women would choose breast-conserving treatment, and that the offer of choice in itself would prevent the significant psychosocial morbidity known to be associated with mastectomy. However, neither of these expectations has been substantiated by the evidence

(Weiss *et al.* 1996; Fallowfield 1997). Another common assumption is that all women with breast cancer wish to participate in the treatment decision-making process (Degner *et al.* 1997), but Chapman *et al.* (1995) caution that individuals probably vary considerably in their appraisal of relevant aspects of the decision.

Shared decision-making aims to facilitate the decision-making process, by educating women about likely outcomes and the supporting evidence, and to involve them in deciding which choice is best (Woolf 1997). In this particular scenario, decisions can be based primarily on patient preferences, as treatment options have comparable outcomes; however, Andrist (1997) points out that individuals will vary regarding both their ability and desire to participate in decision-making. Luker *et al.* (1995) specify that adequate information must be provided or women may feel ill-prepared to take on the role of decision-maker, but although Beaver *et al.* (1996) agree on the importance of information provision, they suggest that not all women will want to make a choice in any case. Charles *et al.* (1997) conclude that information-sharing and treatment decision-making are beginning to be recognized as two separate goals in the medical encounter.

Women's decision-making for mastectomy vs breast-conserving treatment

Various researchers have investigated the decisions women make when offered the choice between mastectomy and breast-conserving treatment, and the factors which influence those decisions. Significant factors described in the literature include: perceptions of physician recommendation, perceptions of disease outcome, importance of body image, prior information, information needs and educational interventions, patient recall, concerns regarding radiotherapy and/or its side-effects, and patient age.

Perceptions of physician recommendation

Woolf (1997) stated that the personal preferences of physicians are irrelevant in this subjective arena, yet women's interpretations of decision-making consultations may differ.

Hughes' exploratory study (1993) of 71 women demonstrated that although treatment choice was not related to any stated physician preference, many subjects reported that their decisions were heavily influenced by physicians' recommendations. Therefore, women's perceptions of physician recommendation, rather than actual physician recommendations, may be significant. The relevance of this issue was also highlighted in a survey of 76 newly diagnosed women by Johnson *et al.* (1996), which found that although 80% of women wanted a role in decision-making, 74% wanted their surgeons to make a recommendation and when given, 94% followed the recommendation. Smitt and Heltzel (1997) concluded from their survey of 261 women, that the physician's recommendation and the patient's perception of chance for cure were the most influential factors affecting treatment decisions.

Perceptions of disease outcome

Hughes (1993) found that some women attributed their treatment decisions to their need to minimize both risk and post-decisional regret, as they interpreted it, rather than to the information which had been provided. Whelan *et al.* (1995) reported that of the 82 participants in their study, women chose breast irradiation to: reduce the risk of a local recurrence, prevent subsequent breast surgery, prevent mastectomy specifically, and to increase survival. In Wei *et al.*'s prospective survey of 300 women (1995), the chance of cancer recurrence affecting choice was significantly different between the groups choosing mastectomy or breast-conserving treatment (88 vs 40%, respectively). It is perhaps significant to note that Wei *et al.*'s research was hypothetical, and that results may differ for women actually diagnosed with breast cancer. However, Weiss *et al.* (1996) also found that despite having been advised to the contrary, most of their 164 patients stated that their chosen treatment—regardless of the option they had chosen—provided the best chance for cure. These studies demonstrate that although health care professionals might consider mastectomy and breast-conserving treatment to be equivalent options, women themselves appear to interpret the situation differently.

Importance of body image

Ward *et al.* (1989) found that nine of the 11 women in their study who chose breast-conserving treatment based their choice on a desire to maintain body integrity. Body integrity was not a significant decision-making factor for the women who chose mastectomy. Wei *et al.* (1995) also reported a difference between mastectomy and lumpectomy groups in the number of women who: thought it important to preserve the breast, and accordingly chose breast-conserving treatment (35 vs 84%), believed too much emphasis had been placed on breast conservation (51 vs 19%), would prefer to keep their own breast (76 vs 96%). There-fore, women's attitudes towards body image and its potential alteration by breast cancer treatment, have a significant influence on the decision-making process.

Prior information

Although much of the decision-making literature focuses on the importance of adequate information provision by health care pro-fessionals, a noteworthy finding from Hughes (1993) was that women's treatment choices were related to information received prior to their consultation, but were not influenced significantly by either the amount of information presented at consultation, or the manner in which it was presented. Hughes also reported that women who chose mastectomy reported receiving information from a greater number of sources than those who chose lumpec-tomy, speculating that women receive less informal information about breast-conserving treatment because it is comparatively new. Most frequently cited sources of prior information were the lay media, relatives and friends, and educational brochures. Hughes (1993) concluded that women's treatment decisions may be biased by early information, regardless of its source, and other researchers have also discussed women's use of informal informa-tion (Griffiths and Leek 1995; Weiss *et al.* 1996).

Richards *et al.* (1995) suggested that women's preferences may be influenced by their attitudes and beliefs based on pre-vious experience, family, friends, the media, and other health pro-fessionals. The potential influence of lay media was also discussed by Black (1995), who conducted an historical survey of women's magazines and found striking similarities between the messages in the early magazines and in older women's breast cancer beliefs today. If further research proves prior information to be a major influence on the decision-making process, health care professionals will need to find ways of accessing and educating the lay population, rather than focusing exclusively on the patient population.

Information needs and educational interventions

A body of recent research has contributed to our understanding of the priority information needs of women with breast cancer. Without exception, the most highly ranked types of information are related to the disease and its treatment (Griffiths and Leek 1995; Luker *et al.* 1995; Meredith *et al.* 1996; Degner *et al.* 1997; Graydon *et al.* 1997). However, as we cannot assume that all women will require the same level of information, Fallowfield (1997) points out that those patients who prefer limited information also deserve due consideration.

Deber (1996) points out that educational interventions are most effective for patients who have an open mind, because once a patient's decision has been made, there is no decision to share. Andrist (1997) agrees that there are no 'immaculate' decisions, with both patients and providers bringing their own beliefs to the scenario. Therefore, not only information priorities, but also patient decision-making preferences, need to be taken into account. As alluded to previously, not all women with breast cancer wish to be active participants in the decision-making process. Beaver *et al.* (1996) reported that of 150 women newly diagnosed with breast cancer, the majority (52%) preferred to play a passive role. The control group preferred a collaborative role (45.5%), indicating that potentially life-threatening situations may make individuals more passive. Fallowfield (1997) agreed, speculating that the perceptions of healthy individuals might differ considerably from those of women actually diagnosed with breast cancer.

Interestingly, Degner *et al.* (1997) reported that only 42% of women overall believed they had achieved their preferred level of control in decision-making, indicating that health care professionals may have considerable work to do in terms of tailoring information to the needs of individual women. Degner *et al.* also found that women surveyed within six months of diagnosis were more likely to believe they had achieved their preferred role than women further from diagnosis, and speculated that either women are becoming assertive, or health care professionals more diligent. Also, worthy of note is as an earlier study of 97 women by Lerman *et al.* (1993) which found that although almost half of the subjects would have preferred greater control over the decision-making process, this factor was unrelated to the development of subsequent psychological distress. While this finding reinforces the complexity of the decision-making process, it cannot be translated as permission to deny women the opportunity of participation.

Various educational interventions have been proposed as methods of increasing patient involvement in the decision-making process. Street *et al.* (1995) stated that such interventions should have at least two aims: first, to legitimize patient participation, as research has demonstrated how the offer of choice in itself might reduce physical and psychological problems (Ashcroft *et al.* 1985; Morris and Ingham 1988; Fallowfield *et al.* 1989); and second, to provide a foundation of accurate information, as it has been suggested that inadequate information may contribute to women's discomfort in adopting an active role in the decision-making process (Luker *et al.* 1995; Beaver *et al.* 1996).

Techniques that can increase patients' understanding of treatment options include drawing pictures, tape recording the consultation, making sure that a support person is also there, providing written information, and using videos to reinforce teaching (Andrist 1997). Educational interventions described in the current literature include written information, audiotapes, videotapes, and, more recently, multimedia packages. Charles *et al.* (1997) describe all such interventions as treatment decision aids, which provide structure for the decision-making process.

Written information

Griffiths and Leek's survey of 141 Oncology Nursing Society (ONS) members and 76 of their patients (Griffiths and Leek 1995) indicated that written information was more effective than other types for both patients and nurses. Unfortunately, a study investigating reading ability among cancer patients demonstrated that only 27% of patients could be expected to understand all of the available written materials (Cooley *et al.* 1995). Degner *et al.* (1997) agree that information is often provided in a form that is simply not understandable for the majority of patients.

Audiotapes and videotapes

Although it has been suggested that some patients may benefit from receiving audiotapes of their consultation and/or information videotapes (Richards *et al.* 1995), their effectiveness compared with other, less expensive resources, has not yet been comprehensively evaluated. Certainly, there appears to be some consumer demand for user-friendly media, and women in one study suggested the use of audio recordings and video information, as well as current literature, to reinforce verbal information (Bottomley 1997).

Multimedia packages

There has been a recent increase in patient-oriented educational technologies such as interactive multimedia programs that allow the patient to choose which topics to view (Chapman *et al.* 1995; Street *et al.* 1995).

Although educational interventions may be valuable complements to verbal communication, they are not substitutes for individual, person-to-person consultations. Both nurses and patients (Griffiths and Leek 1995) reported that one-on-one conversations about cancer are the most effective source of information, and Bilodeau and Degner (1996) also found that personal sources of information were most important to women.

Problems associated with the use of educational interventions include: provision of equivalent adequate information for those women who do not speak English (Griffiths and Leek 1995) or those with some form of learning difficulty, ensuring that the level of information is appropriate for individual patients, tailoring general information to an individual patient scenario, and finding adequate time to use the materials.

Patient recall

Even where health care providers make concerted efforts to provide appropriate and adequate information to women making breast cancer treatment choices, evidence suggests that patient recall may be seriously impaired. Fallowfield (1997) states that:

'information needs to be given systematically, at the right time and via several different routes, to maximise the chances for patients to understand the implications and make really informed choices'.

However, the 'right time' for patients may not be the most opportune time for the health care professionals.

Cimprich (1993) pointed out that information-giving for women with breast cancer is often limited to around the time of diagnosis, despite evidence indicating that attention and recall are severely limited in life-threatening situations. Hughes (1993) found that 6–8 weeks post-operatively, 48% of women who chose breast-conserving treatment could only recall one of 13 information items presented during their consultation, and 66% of the mastectomy group were unable to recall a single item of the 10 presented. The 26 women in Palsson and Norberg's study (1995) described how difficult it was to participate in decision-making immediately after receiving their diagnosis. Interesting to note, however, is that in Weiss *et al.*'s study (1996), only a small number of women would have preferred more time to make a decision, and under 2% would retrospectively have preferred a different treatment.

Although the role of information in decision-making is widely acknowledged, any direct influence on women's decision-making preferences or treatment choices remains uncertain. Street *et al.* (1995) reported that although women assigned to either an interactive multimedia program or brochure subsequently demonstrated an improved understanding of breast cancer treatment (more so with the multimedia program), their level of participation in the decision-making process was unaffected. Similarly, Chapman *et al.* (1995) found that while videotapes and booklets both increased knowledge scores, knowledge gains were uncorrelated with treatment preferences. The authors did observe a preference shift toward breast-conserving treatment for 69 of 81 subjects who viewed the videotape, but accounted for this finding by noting that some features of the video were not reproduced in the booklet (patient interviews). The subjects in Chapman *et al.*'s study were undergraduate students acting as advisors to a hypothetical patient; therefore, it is difficult to know whether similar results would be seen in women with a breast cancer diagnosis.

Whelan *et al.* (1995) developed a Decision Board (DB) to provide women with detailed information regarding breast cancer treatment options, thus facilitating the decision-making process. Specific aspects of knowledge were improved for the 30 subjects following consultation with the DB, and women's perception of being offered a choice was greater (97 vs 70%). 81% of women who used the DB stated that it helped them think of further questions to ask, and 67% reported showing the DB to someone else. Interestingly, women who used the DB rated physician's recommendation as less influential in their decision, indicating that improved knowledge perhaps influenced their confidence in assuming some responsibility for decision-making. However, although 81% of patients using the DB felt that it helped them make a decision, it did not alter their subsequent choice of treatment, as determined by comparison with the control group.

Concerns regarding radiotherapy and/or its side-effects

Ward *et al.* (1989) found that concerns about radiotherapy were significantly different for women choosing breast conservation over mastectomy, with women choosing mastectomy because of concerns about the efficacy of radiotherapy (9/11), and/or worries about the side-effects or inconvenience of radiotherapy (7/11). Subsequent studies have also found concerns about radiotherapy to have a significant influence on treatment decisions.

Wei *et al.* (1995) demonstrated that there was no difference in the number of women choosing mastectomy versus breast-conserving treatment who expressed a fear of radiation generally (60 vs 63%). However, of the women who had selected mastectomy, a significant number had a fear of radiation therapy (76 vs 57%) and of the side-effects (80 vs 63%). Other authors have also demonstrated the importance of patient's perceptions of potential side-effects (Meredith *et al.* 1996; Smitt and Heltzel 1997). Most patients in Bottomley's study, 72% of whom were waiting to commence radiotherapy, reported that they were afraid of the treatment they would receive (Bottomley 1997).

Side-effects of adjuvant radiotherapy for early breast cancer can be classified as early or late:

Early side-effects begin during or shortly after treatment, are temporary, and usually last for up to a month following treatment (Bates and Evans 1995). These commonly include fatigue, oedema, breast tenderness, and skin reactions (Engelking and Kalinowski 1995). Fatigue is the commonest symptom reported by patients receiving radiotherapy, affecting self-care and social activities (Oberst *et al.* 1991; Longman *et al.* 1997; Hoskins 1997). Although loss of appetite, reddening or blistering of the irradiated skin, temporary difficulty in swallowing, and nausea and vomiting may occur, these side-effects are rare (Bates and Evans 1995).

Late side-effects begin weeks, months, or years after treatment, tend to persist, and to become progressively worse (Bates and Evans 1995). These mainly affect tissues within the radiotherapy treatment field, including skin, cardiac tissue, nerve tissue, and bone. Skin changes include telangiectasia, dyspigmentation, and very occasionally chronic ulceration of the skin; however, these are rare with modern techniques unless the skin has been deliberately irradiated as part of the treatment plan. Likewise, technical advances have minimized cardiac exposure to radiation (Abrams *et al.* 1995), and a study by Rutqvist *et al.* (1998) found no indication of an increased acute myocardial infarction risk with breast-conserving treatment. Abrams *et al.* (1995) also stated that radiation-induced second cancers should not be a factor in treatment decisions, due to their rarity.

There has been considerable publicity in recent years regarding severe late side-effects following radiotherapy, particularly brachial plexus neuropathy. Following requests from the group Radiation Action Group Exposure (RAGE), an independent review was commissioned by the Royal College of Radiologists (Bates and Evans 1995). This review described severe late side-effects experienced by 126 of 249 members of RAGE who were treated at a number of cancer centres during the 14-year period 1980–1993, and who agreed to cooperate. Problems experienced by the women in this group included brachial plexus neuropathy (BPN) (38%), sometimes leading to development of a useless arm; pain (71% of those women with BPN); subcutaneous fibrosis leading to a painful stiff shoulder and/or a deformed breast (46%);

bone necrosis often resulting in fractures of ribs or clavicle (14%); and lymphoedema of the arm (37%). Bates and Evans (1995) concluded that although women studied in the report had certainly suffered as a result of radiation damage, these women were not generally representative of the estimated 65 000 women treated at the specified cancer centres during the time period reviewed. The authors stressed the importance of stating that such serious side-effects following radiotherapy for early operable breast cancer are not usual, particularly now that technical advances have significantly minimized risks.

As stated previously, women's perceptions of the inconvenience incurred by attending radiotherapy treatment ranks highly as a decision-making criteria. Abrams *et al.* (1995) stated that patients and physicians should take factors such as travel time into account, as part of the decision-making process. Correspondingly, Wei *et al.* (1995) demonstrated that there was no difference in the number of women choosing mastectomy versus breast-conserving treatment who felt that attending outpatient radiotherapy would impose a family hardship on them (51 vs 48%). There was no difference in travelling distances reported by the groups; however, more women in the mastectomy group stated that the issue of five weeks of radiotherapy would sway their selection of treatment (51 vs 33%). In practical terms, although 64% of the 252 oncology outpatients in Thomas *et al.*'s (1997) study reported that transport was 'no problem at all', and a further 25% reported that it was 'relatively easy', difficulties were experienced by 11% of patients, most of whom had to be transported by ambulance, taxi, or driven by friends or relatives. Women in Bottomley's study (1997) discussed their frustration regarding lack of control over transport and the distance travelled, and financial cost was also raised as a significant transport issue.

Age

Although some studies have indicated that older women may be less concerned with altered body image than their younger counterparts, Hughes (1993) found that older women were not any more likely to choose mastectomy versus breast-conserving treatment. Likewise, Meyer *et al.* (1995) reported that although older women sought less information when making treatment decisions, and made their decisions faster, the treatment choices made were equivalent to those of younger women. Furthermore, 65% of women who made immediate decisions, did not change their minds when given more information. Meyer *et al.* described how older women focused on the need for a decision 'before the cancer had time to spread', whereas younger women focused on the need for more information. Degner *et al.* (1997) found that women younger than 50 years ranked physical and sexual attractiveness as more important than their older counterparts, and older women rated information about self-care as more important; however, information priorities do not necessarily determine treatment choices.

The discussion presented above has focused mainly on the role of the patient in the breast cancer treatment decision-making process, and on the factors influencing the patient's role. However, while a patient-oriented approach is undoubtedly justifiable, Lerman *et al.* (1993) caution that the responsibility for communication and/or communication problems must not be placed solely with the patient. Therefore it is necessary also to consider the role of other participants in the decision-making process. Meredith *et al.* (1996) propose that as individual health care professionals often focus on different aspects of patient's needs, and patients themselves often share different concerns or information to each discipline, more comprehensive care can be provided by multidisciplinary collaboration. Although many individuals may contribute to each woman's decision-making process, those currently acknowledged in the literature are physicians, nurses, and family and friends.

The physician

Patients' satisfaction with their physician has been shown to eclipse all other patient satisfaction variables (Grogan *et al.* 1995). Furthermore, Thomas *et al.* (1995) noted that seeing the same doctor at each clinic visit was considered to be important, especially for relatively new patients, with the importance of seeing the consultant, specifically, considered to be slightly less important overall. Unfortunately, Charles *et al.* (1997) point out that several physicians are often involved in the decision-making process with a single patient, although the impact of continuity— or lack of it—is not explicitly described in the literature. This issue is perhaps especially pertinent for women who undergo definitive surgery in a district general hospital, and are then referred to a cancer centre for radiotherapy treatment, consequently having to establish relationships with two geographically distant sets of health care professionals.

Although the pivotal role of the physician is undisputed, various authors have discussed difficulties with the patient/doctor interaction. In Lerman *et al.*'s study (1993), 84% of breast cancer patients reported difficulties communicating with the medical team, and while the severity of problems reported was relatively low, they were more common among patients who were less optimistic about their disease and had less assertive coping styles, possibly identifying a group of particularly vulnerable individuals in the treatment decision-making scenario. The authors commented that although providers offered information and explanations, many patients had problems comprehending this information, asking questions, and expressing their own feelings. Worthy of some concern are the findings of Ford *et al.* (1994), who assessed five oncologists and demonstrated that although recognition of psychological distress is a crucial aspect of patient care, clinicians tended to under-rate distress exhibited by their patients, and were mostly satisfied with their own performance during consultations. Exploring the decision-making scenario from the patient's perspective, Johnson *et al.* (1996) reported that of women who had specific fears (76% of the 76 women surveyed), only half revealed such fears to their doctor, and consequently, 45% of women had their fears unrecognized. If further research demonstrates that women have significant difficulties in communicating effectively with their physicians, they are unlikely to be comfortable with participation in the decision-making process.

Bottomley (1997) and Woolf (1997) discuss how patients' perceptions of doctors, particularly surgeons, as 'very busy', inhibits the patient/doctor interaction. Although Woolf suggested that physicians who lack time can send patients home with materials or can delegate some steps to other colleagues, Meredith *et al.* (1996) reported that the majority of patients (60%) in their study preferred to discuss their cancer with their hospital specialist.

Social class, gender, age, race, and ethnicity are all acknowledged as playing a part in the interaction between physician and
patient (Andrist 1997). However, Feldman *et al.* (1997) and
McKinlay *et al.* (1997) investigated the role of 'non-medical'
influences on clinical decision-making behaviour, and both studies concluded that numerous intangible factors are also involved.
Meredith *et al.* (1996) concluded that in order to achieve optimal
benefit for patients, doctors need sufficient time and appropriate
surroundings, as well as knowledge, understanding, and good
clinical skills.

The nurse

Nurses usually spend more time with patients than their physicians and develop a relationship that facilitates patient communication (Kedziera and Levy 1994). Accordingly, Griffiths and Leek
(1995) suggest that the nurse/patient relationship is an important
and powerful resource on which to capitalize. Although nurses
may be perceived by the lay public as having a mainly 'hands
on' physical caring role, Krishnasamy's small pilot study (1996)
indicated that emotionally supportive behaviour patterns are the
most frequently identified, helpful nurse interactions for patients
with cancer, followed by informationally supportive behaviours.
Thomas *et al.* (1997) and Bottomley (1997) reported that cancer
patients typically saw nurses in a supportive role, as friend,
confidante, explainer, comforter, counsellor, as well as nurse.
Furthermore, nurses in Thomas *et al.*'s study were perceived by
patients as providing continuity of care when patients did not
always see the same physician.

In terms of the treatment decision-making scenario, various
authors have discussed the role of the nurse as a facilitator, assisting women in formulating questions, assessing preferred level of
participation, clarifying and reinforcing information, and liaising
with medical colleagues where appropriate (Luker *et al.* 1995;
Richards *et al.* 1995; Bilodeau and Degner 1996). However,
Luker *et al.* (1995) advise that these responsibilities may fall
within the remit of the clinical nurse specialist in breast care,
rather than being within the scope of the average ward nurse.

Fallowfield (1997) agrees that the advent of the clinical nurse specialist appears to be a step in the right direction but cautions that nursing, as with other interventions, is worthy of more thorough evaluation.

Family and friends

In addition to survival predictions and potential side-effects of treatment, patients and physicians should also consider the role of social support (Oberst *et al.* 1991; Abrams *et al.* 1995), and Oberst *et al.* (1991) suggested that those patients without a supportive social support network might need additional support during treatment. Certainly, Richards *et al.* (1995) and Bottomley (1997) highlighted the value of friends and relatives as emotional supporters, and Meredith *et al.* (1996) discussed the significance of establishing relationships with other women, newly diagnosed with breast cancer. However, in addition to the invaluable emotionally supportive role, Charles *et al.* (1997) suggest that family members or friends can play the roles of information gatherer, recorder or interpreter, coach/prompt, advisor, negotiator, and caretaker in the treatment decision-making process.

Hughes (1993) demonstrated that for women with early breast cancer, family and friends were frequently cited as sources of prior information, which in turn was related to treatment choices. Bilodeau and Degner (1996) found that women approached friends or relatives for information slightly more frequently than they approached nurses, and Smitt and Heltzel (1997) stated that the majority of women in their study consulted only with the surgeon (96%), primary care physician (64%), and spouse (75% among married patients), before making a treatment choice. These findings imply that family and friends of women offered a choice of treatments for breast cancer have an important role to play in the decision-making process, with patient preferences potentially influenced by family and friends (Richards *et al.* 1995). However, Charles *et al.* (1997) point out that the current literature relating to shared decision-making focuses almost exclusively on the dyad relationship of physician and patient.

Implications for health care professionals

Ream and Richardson (1996) conducted a literature review to explore the role of information in facilitating cancer patients' adaptation to treatment. The authors concluded that therapeutic relationships are maximized when medical and nursing staff correctly assess and fulfil the individual information requirements of their patients. In terms of the breast cancer treatment decision-making scenario specifically, Beaver *et al.* (1996) state that health professionals need to systematically assess each woman's preferences for participation in treatment decisions. Charles *et al.* (1997) point out, however, that information-sharing does not necessarily lead to a sharing of the treatment decision-making process, and Woolf (1997) agrees that the intent is not to force patients to make decisions, but to give them the opportunity to participate. Therefore, the challenge for health professionals is not to devise one decision-making package or intervention, but to be flexible in their approach to each woman, assessing individual needs and preferences, and exploring the diverse factors which might influence her decision.

New developments in the use of radiotherapy for breast cancer

The majority of current research focuses on the use of radiotherapy as a local treatment for early breast cancer; however, recent studies suggest that local radiotherapy may also have systemic benefits. Although the Early Breast Cancer Trialists' Collaborative Group (1995) overview of 36 randomized trials suggested only a limited benefit from radiotherapy in terms of breast-cancer mortality, a number of recently published trials have found that adjuvant radiotherapy not only reduces the risk of local recurrence, but also lowers the risk of subsequent distant metastasis (Arriagada *et al.* 1995; Forrest *et al.* 1996; Overgaard *et al.* 1997; Ragaz *et al.* 1997). Yarnold (1997) points out that this systemic benefit had been suggested by trials conducted in the prechemotherapy era, but any potential reduction in breast cancer mortality was offset by the risk of fatal radiation-related cardiac disease with techniques in use at that time. Further clinical trials are likely to be conducted to identify specific subgroups of women who will gain worthwhile benefits from postmastectomy radiotherapy.

The way forward

Although there is a growing body of literature related to decision-making generally, and to breast cancer treatment decision-making specifically, very few of the studies discussed in this chapter meet the scientific rigour expected of contemporary clinical research. Therefore, there is not yet sufficient evidence on which to base clinical practice.

Future research needs to:

- compare the effectiveness of various educational interventions in specific subgroups of women
- consider the role of prior/informal information in women's decision-making
- explore whether women's attitudes toward radiotherapy will change over generations, as breast-conserving treatment becomes better known
- examine the psychological effects, in terms of anxiety and depression, of women's varying levels of involvement in decision-making
- evaluate the contributions of various members of the multidisciplinary team, and family and friends, to the decision-making scenario.

Radiotherapy—a personal perspective

Helen

The radiotherapy, people said, was the final hurdle—get through that and then life could start returning to normal. In fact I didn't really give it very much thought—after everything else I'd been through, it seemed much the least daunting of the three stages of treatment. I'd pondered a great deal about the what ifs of both surgery and chemotherapy. Since my diagnosis I'd scoured the medical journals and shamelessly exploited my medical friends to double check that I'd grasped concepts and terminology. I'd also made it plain that assimilating information about my illness, asking questions, and obtaining answers that didn't gloss over the ambiguities and complexities were all an essential part of my coping mechanism. It had been traumatic as an extremely fit 42-year-old to learn I'd got breast cancer but once diagnosed, I was determined to understand as much as I could about the disease and the variables that applied in my own case.

The chemotherapy had turned out to be much less of an ordeal than I'd imagined—yes I'd felt pretty awful for a couple of days after treatment but I'd carried on working throughout and the sessions themselves had been rather jolly sociable occasions—lots of activity, banter, and cups of tea. Going for chemo was an event to which friends volunteered to come along. Amazingly, when you got to the IV room you also came across the same people who'd treated you three weeks before, and they remembered things that you'd said when you were there the last time. There was a continuity of medical staff at a point when you most needed it; added to this was the fact that there were rarely more than three or four patients being dealt with at the same time. So tough as it was, in many respects the experience was at a personal, individual level, profoundly affirming.

Another five weeks or so for the radiotherapy and the whole thing would be over. Having to visit the hospital every day for half an hour or so for this last stretch did not seem particularly arduous and was something I felt I could accommodate without too much disruption to my working day. I realize now that I underestimated just how tired I was. Continuing to work throughout my treatment had been in many ways extremely positive, but it had created a frame of mind in which it was difficult for me to admit that perhaps I needed a break. As things turned out, the radiotherapy was for me the most gruelling part of all my treatment.

On my first visit to the unit, the registrar went over my details and asked would I be interested in taking part in a randomized trial—whereby I might end up either having a higher dose for a shorter period of three weeks or the standard dose over five to seven weeks. I'd made it clear from the start that I was happy to participate in trials and had willingly participated in the Clodroplac trial earlier, which was also randomized. This time, however, I simply wasn't interested. I assumed a higher dose might mean a greater likelihood of irritation and I was anyway concerned about the possibility of oedema—wouldn't there be a higher risk of this with a higher dosage over a shorter period? Normally, I would have asked questions and then made my decision whether to participate or not, but by now I was too tired to bother with yet more questions. I said I'd prefer to opt for the standard course of treatment over five weeks and not take part in the trial. I felt somewhat guilty about this decision, even though the registrar made it absolutely clear there was no pressure to participate.

Up to this point, I felt I had coped extremely well with the aftermath of both surgery and chemotherapy but now I was feeling much more emotionally vulnerable. I can still recall quite early on in the radiotherapy treatment, being positioned on the trolley in the usual way, and as everyone rushed behind the screen and I struggled to remain as still as possible while the dose was being given, finding involuntary tears streaming down my face. The relentless daily grind of getting to the hospital, the hanging around, the sense of isolation as the treatment was being given, compounded by the increasing exhaustion as the treatment progressed, all contributed to making this last phase much harder to deal with than I had anticipated.

Through reading, research, and the help of sympathetic medical staff, I'd managed to understand some of the issues and considerations involved in making treatment decisions concerning surgery and, in the case of chemotherapy, had been engaged in an active discussion about options. With radiotherapy, however, it felt as if there were no options—or at least none that the patient could meaningfully be involved in. The whole process was also so driven by technology that it seemed impossible get to grips with it. Despite the fact that both the radiotherapy team and the senior medical staff I dealt with were exceptionally helpful, informative, and kind, basically it felt that once the dosage had been calculated, one was in a system where the primary aim was to get you through as quickly and efficiently as possible.

It felt as if there was a lot more waiting around involved with the radiotherapy—machines seemed to regularly break down or be in need of servicing and staff would be frantically trying to reschedule patients in order to fit every one in. I soon learnt that the later in the day the appointment, the more likely and longer the hold-ups. Despite the faultless good humour of the staff in dealing with all this, it was difficult not to feel frustrated by the delays followed by what was literally just 30 seconds of treatment. I regarded myself as a pretty resilient patient and I had been treated supremely well by all the medical staff I met, but despite this, I was surprised at how stressful by this stage I was finding the whole business of coming into the hospital on a daily basis.

For me, radiotherapy was at the end of a long line of treatment. I was extremely tired, I felt unqualified to take any view on what was happening to me, and at times it felt as if the factory-like nature of the process—despite the best efforts of the staff involved—left one with little sense of individuality within the system. I should stress that the sensitivity and good humour of the radiotherapy teams was equal to anything I encountered elsewhere in my treatment but nevertheless, as a patient, I felt quite isolated during this final part of treatment.

I'm not sure what could have been done that would have countered this. Possibly greater continuity of breast care nursing support into the radiotherapy phase of treatment? This had, in my own case, been extremely valuable in helping me cope with surgery and chemotherapy. Maybe because of the premium I attached to having access to information, I had assumed that this was what I would need at every stage of treatment including radiotherapy. Whereas by this point, it was less hard information I wanted but more the opportunity, every now and again, to discuss how I was feeling. What I now realize is how, in the earlier stages of treatment, particularly during chemotherapy, much of that side of things had been managed through the informal day-to-day relationship with nursing staff. Whereas, when it came to radiotherapy, the nature of the process meant there were fewer opportunities for this kind of informal support—however willing the staff involved might have been to offer it. On the basis of my own experience, I would say that, while radiotherapy was part of an overall continuum of patient care, it did feel different in kind from the previous stages of treatment and that it is perhaps easy to underestimate the type and amount of emotional support required to help the patient through this phase.

14

Resource organizations

Breast Cancer Care

Breast Cancer Care is a national organization offering free information, help, and support to those affected by breast cancer and other breast-related problems. Betty Westgate set up the charity in 1973. She had recently had a mastectomy and wanted to relieve other women of some of the loneliness and distress she had experienced. Their services are free, confidential, and accessible to all.

The Breast Cancer Care Helpline

The Helpline provides information and support and aims to enable callers to make choices that are right for them. Breast care nurses and volunteers, many of whom have personal experience of breast cancer, staff the Helpline. All staff have been trained in listening skills, and can give emotional support, practical advice, and medical information. Call the Helpline free and in confidence on 0500 245345 Monday–Friday 10 am–5 pm.

The volunteer service

Many women who have breast cancer or breast-related problems find it helps to talk to someone who has shared a similar experience. Breast Cancer Care has volunteers across the country who have all had personal experience of breast cancer or benign breast disease. All our volunteers are trained to provide emotional support to anyone diagnosed with breast cancer or worried about benign breast disease. Many of our volunteers are women under 45. The volunteer service has a network of younger women that younger patients can talk to. We also have male volunteers with a diagnosis of breast cancer with whom male patients can be put in touch. In addition, Breast Cancer Care has partner volunteers. It can be very difficult coming to terms with the news that your partner has breast cancer and partners may need support for themselves. You can ask for a volunteer at any stage of treatment or recovery by telephoning the Breast Cancer Care Helpline 0500 245345.

The information service

Breast Cancer Care provides a range of free publications related to breast awareness and breast cancer. Information is also available about local self-help groups and other organizations that might be helpful. For more information call the Breast Cancer Care Helpline on 0500 245345.

The prosthesis fitting service

The free prosthesis fitting service has been developed over many years to give a sensitive, personal, and professional service for women who need practical advice and help after breast surgery. They hold an extensive range of prostheses from seven manufacturers in all sizes and all skin tones. They also stock a range of non-pocket bras and mastectomy swimsuits. For NHS patients they can help you choose a prosthesis that you can obtain from your hospital free of charge. And for non-NHS and overseas customers they provide a full sales service too.

For an appointment call 0171 384 2984 (London) or 0141 353 1050 (Glasgow or Edinburgh).

CancerBACUP (formerly known as BACUP)

CancerBACUP is a leading national charity providing information, counselling, and support for people with cancer, their families, and friends. It also provides services for health professionals. Its Cancer Support Service is staffed by specialist cancer nurses and professional counsellors. CancerBACUP has the full backing of patient groups. It publishes 51 booklets on specific cancers, treatments, and on living with cancer. All services are provided free of charge and in confidence to anyone affected by cancer.

CancerBACUP, 3 Bath Place, Rivington Street, London EC2A 3JR. Counselling: 0171 696 9000.

CancerBACUP Scotland, 30 Bell Street, Glasgow G1 ILG. Tel: 0141 553 1553 (Monday–Friday 9 am–5.30 pm). Information: 0800 181199 (Monday–Friday 9 am–7 pm). Minicom textphone available.

Cancerlink

Cancerlink provides information and emotional support in response to telephone enquiries and letters on all aspects of cancer to people with cancer, their families, friends, carers, and professionals working with them. It acts as a resource to around 600 cancer self-help and support groups nationwide and can put people in touch with their local groups. Groups vary in size and remit and there are a number which focus on breast cancer and the issues it evokes. A range of publications about cancer and the emotional and practical issues about living with cancer are available on request.

Cancerlink, 11–21 Northdown Street, London N1 9BN. Admin: 0171 833 2818; Fax: 0171 833 4963.

0800 132905	Freephone Cancer Information Helpline (Monday–Friday 9.30 am–1 pm, 2–5 pm)
0800 591028	Freephone MAC Helpline for young people (Monday–Friday 9.30 am–1 pm, 2–5 pm)
0800 590415	Freephone Asian Cancer Information Helpline in Bengali, Hindi, English, Punjabi and Urdu) (Monday 10 am–1 pm, Friday 10 am–1 pm, 2–4 pm)

The Irish Cancer Society

The Irish Cancer Society is the national cancer charity dedicated to eliminating cancer by preventing cancer, saving lives from cancer, and improving the quality of life of those who develop cancer by patient care, education, and research.

Care—The Irish Cancer Society provides a free Cancer Helpline staffed by specially trained nurses who are available to offer help, information, and advice. 'Phone 1800 200 700.

Reach to Recovery—is a helpful and supportive programme for women who are about to have, or who have recently had, breast surgery. The programme works on the principle of personal contact between the patient and a Reach to Recovery volunteer—herself a woman who has had breast surgery. Carefully selected and fully trained volunteers are available to provide advice and reassurance at a time when the patient is in most need of both.

Education and Information—The Society's Health Promotion Department provides lectures, seminars, and workshops to women's groups, organizations, and to workplaces on all aspects of breast cancer—early detection screening and recovery.

Detailed leaflets are available free of charge under the following titles: *Breast Cancer—What you should know; Breast Self Examination; Understanding Breast Cancer* (patient information booklet).

The Cancer Research Advancement Board (CRAB) is an autonomous body within a framework of the Irish Cancer Society and is responsible for evaluating research proposals for funding research programmes. CRAB seeks to ensure that funded programmes are directly relevant to the Irish situation and are aimed at improving patient diagnosis, treatment, and management in Ireland. Breast cancer research is financed through this Board.

The Irish Cancer Society, 5 Northumberland Rd, Dublin 4, Ireland. Tel: 01 668 1855; Fax: 01 668 7599; Email: admin@irishcancer.ie.

Macmillan Cancer Relief

Macmillan Cancer Relief, in partnership with others, contributes to a number of initiatives and services provided to families with a diagnosis of breast cancer. Macmillan's aim is to develop and promote new ideas for treatment and care of cancer patients and their families which will make their lives easier and reduce unnecessary levels of fear.

Breast cancer is a complex disease and women need reliable information in order to understand treatments and to decide what is right for them. The provision of information is essential to ensure that women are assisted to make the right decisions for them and to enable them to give informed consent.

Macmillan in association with others ran a Breast Cancer Awareness Campaign in 1996. Two leaflet were produced *A Guide to Common Breast Problems* and *Breast Cancer—How to Help Yourself*. The latter provides 10 minimum standards for care of the patient facing a diagnosis of breast cancer.

It is common that patients, when being given their diagnosis, have been scared to ask the questions they want to ask, however well prepared they were. It is common for patients to retain little of the information about, for example, prognosis or treatment options in response to the type of issues and others.

Macmillan Cancer Relief has responded to this need through pump priming 150 Macmillan clinical nurse specialists in breast care since 1988. The prime purpose of these posts is to provide a continuing support service from the point of diagnosis throughout hospital and community care to patients with breast cancer and their families. The focus of the post is to provide direct or indirect assistance to the patient throughout their management, particularly improving support, patient education, counselling, and advice. Working as members of the multidisciplinary team, they have additional activities of clinical intervention; for example, they are required to develop practice, to disseminate best practice, and to provide a resource and educationalist role for other health care professionals.

For further information on Macmillan's activities call the Macmillan Information Line on 0845 601 6161. Macmillan Cancer Relief, National Office, Anchor House, 15–19 Britten Street, London, SW3 3TZ. Administration: 0171 351 7811; Fax: 0171 376 8098.

TAK TENT—Cancer Support Scotland

Tak Tent Cancer Support Scotland is one of the 500 or so self-help organizations in the UK that enable patients, their relatives, and friends to find appropriate help and support to cope emotionally and psychologically with the impact of the diagnosis and treatment of cancer.

The organization has a network of 17 groups in local communities, largely in the west of Scotland, offering mutual support. Each meets monthly, with individual help and counselling provided from the Resource Centre in Glasgow and on the telephone Helpline.

The organization helps anyone affected by cancer, including a large number facing the diagnosis and treatment of breast cancer. All the work is person-centred, responding to the needs of those who seek help. Those who wish to speak with fellow patients, relatives, or friends are put in touch, and whenever appropriate, referrals are also made to other related organizations. Those aged 16–25 years old are linked to the Youth Project.

Tak Tent Office, The Western Infirmary, Block 20 Western Court, 100 University Place, Glasgow, G12 6SQ. Resource Centre: 0141 211 1932; Admin: 0141 211 1930; Fax: 0141 211 1879.

Tenovus Cancer Information Centre

The Tenovus Cancer Information Centre provides information and support in response to telephone enquiries and letters on all aspects of cancer to people with cancer, their families, friends, carers, and professionals working with them. A range of free information publications, both booklets and leaflets, is available on request. The free national Helpline is answered by trained nurses.

Tenovus Cancer Information Centre, PO Box 88, College Buildings, Courtney Rd, Splott, Cardiff CF1 1SA. Freephone Cancer Information Helpline: 0800 526 527; Admin: 01222 49770; Fax: 01222 489919.

The Ulster Cancer Foundation

The Ulster Cancer Foundation is a charity providing a wide range of services for women affected by breast cancer and their families in Northern Ireland.

A Freephone Cancer Helpline (0800 783 3339) is available Monday–Friday 9 am–5 pm. This is staffed by specially trained cancer nurses with experience in counselling. From the first symptoms throughout the course of their illness, information, support, and counselling are at hand for patients, their families, and carers.

As women face the prospect of surgery for their breast cancer, they are offered a visit from a volunteer befriender. These are women who have had breast cancer themselves, have been successfully treated, and have adjusted well. The volunteers are carefully selected and trained by the Foundation. Some volunteers are trained to run the Foundation's fitting service which provides suitable underwear and swimwear for women who have had breast surgery.

Thirteen Breast Cancer Support Groups are run throughout the province. These meet on a regular basis to provide ongoing support for women living with breast cancer and their families.

The Foundation also works for new and better treatments for cancer, as well as helping young people and adults to reduce the risk of developing the disease.

The Ulster Cancer Foundation, 40/42 Eglantine Avenue, Belfast BT9 6DX. Freephone Cancer Information Helpline: 0800 7833339; Admin: 01232 663281; Fax: 01232 660081.

References

Abrams, J.S., Phillips, P.H., and Friedman, M.A. (1995). Meeting highlights: a reappraisal of research results for the local treatment of early stage breast cancer. *Journal of the National Cancer Institute*, **87**, 1837–45.

Alderson, P., Maddon, M., Oakley, A., and Wilkins, R. (1994). *Women's views of breast cancer treatment and research: report of pilot project 1993*. Social Science Research Unit, University of London, London.

Andersson, M., Storm, H., and Mouridsen, H. (1991). Incidence of new primary cancer after adjuvant tamoxifen and radiotherapy for early breast cancer. *Journal of the National Cancer Institute*, **83**, 1013–17.

Andrist, L. (1997). A feminist model for women's health care. *Nursing Inquiry*, **4**, 268–74.

Ardern-Jones, A. (1997). *Living with a cancer legacy*. MSc thesis, University of London, London.

Aristotle, c.340 BC. *The Nicomachean Ethics of Aristotle* (trans. and introd. W.D. Ross). Oxford University Press, London, 1959.

Arriagada, R., Rutqvist, L.E., Mattsson, A., Kramar, A., and Rotstein, S. (1995). Adequate locoregional treatment for early breast cancer may prevent secondary dissemination. *Journal of Clinical Oncology*, **13**, 2869–78.

Ashcroft, J.J., Leinster, S.J., and Glade, P.D. (1985). Breast cancer-patient choice of treatment: preliminary communication. *Journal of Royal Society of Medicine*, **78**, 43–6.

Audit Commission (1993). *What seems to be the matter: communication between hospitals and patients*. HMSO, London.

Austoker, J. (1997). *Breast cancer screening*, Factsheet 7. Cancer Research Campaign.

Austoker, J. and Patnick, J. (ed.), (1993). Report of the UKCCCR/ NHSBSP workshop: *Breast screening acceptability, research, and practice*. NHSBSP Publications No. 28.

Barry, M.J., Floyd, J., Fowler, J.R., Mulley, A.G., Henderson, J.V., and Wennberg, M. D. (1995). Patient reaction to a program designed to facilitate patient participation in treatment decisions for benign prostatic hyperplasia. *Medical Care*, **33**, 771–82.

Baskerville, P., Heddle, R., and Jarrett, P. (1985). Preparation of surgery: information tapes for the patient. *Practitioner*, **229**, 677–88.

Bates, T. and Evans, R.G.B. (1995). *Report of the Independent Review commissioned by the Royal College of Radiologists into brachial plexus neuropathy following radiotherapy for breast carcinoma*. The Royal College of Radiologists, London.

Baum, M. (1982). *Breast cancer lessons from the past*, 1, 649–60.

Baum, M. (1986). Do we need informed consent? *Lancet*, Oct. 18, 911–2.

Baum, M. (1990). Trends in primary breast cancer management, where are we going? *Surgical Clinics of North America*, 70, 1187–92.

Baum, M. (1994). Clinical trials—a brave new partnership: a response to Mrs Thornton. *Journal of Medical Ethics*, 20, 23–5.

Baum, M. (1995a). The ethics of randomised controlled trials. *European Journal of Surgical Oncology*, 21, 136–9.

Baum, M. (1995b). The ethics of clinical trials. *Israel Journal of Medical Science*, 31, 197–200.

Baum, M., and Houghton, J. (1988). Informed consent and controlled trials. *Lancet*, Nov. 19, 1194.

Baum, M., Zilkha, K., and Houghton, J. (1989). Ethics of clinical research: lessons for the future. *British Medical Journal*, 299, 251–3.

Baum, M., Saunders, C., and Meredith, S. (1994). *Breast cancer, a guide for every woman*. Oxford University Press.

Beauchamp, T. and Childress, J. (1994). *Principles of biomedical ethics*. Oxford University Press.

Beaver, K., Luker, K.A., Owens, R.G., Leinster, S.J., Degner, L.F., and Sloane, J.A. (1996). Treatment decision making in women newly diagnosed with breast cancer. *Cancer Nursing*, 19, 8–19.

Beisecker, A.E. and Beisecker, T.D. (1990). Patient information-seeking behaviours when communicating with doctors. *Medical Care*, 28, 19–28.

Belmont Report (1978). *National commission for the protection of human subjects and biomedical and behavioural research*. DHEW Publications, 578–001, pp. 4–8. US Government Printing Office, Washington DC.

Benner, P. and Wrubel, J. (1989). *The primacy of caring*. Addison-Wesley, California.

Benson, J. (1983). Who is the autonomous man? *Philosophy*, 58, 5–17.

Bentham, J. (1948). Introduction to the principles of morals and legislation. In *Fragment on government and introduction to the principles of morals and legislation*, (ed. W. Harrison). Blackwell, Oxford.

Bergh, J. (1997). Time for integration of predictive factors for selection of breast cancer patients who need postoperative radiation therapy? *Journal of the National Cancer Institute*, 89, 605–7.

Bilodeau, B. and Degner, L. (1996). Information needs, sources of information, and decisional roles in women with breast cancer. *Oncology Nursing Forum*, 23, 691–6.

Bird, A.W. (1994). Enhancing patient well-being: advocacy or negotiation? *Journal of Medical Ethics*, **20**, 152–6.

Black, M.E.A. (1995). What did popular women's magazines from 1929 to 1949 say about breast cancer? *Cancer Nursing*, **18**, 270–7.

Blanchard, C.G., Labrecque, M.S., Ruckdeschel, J.C., and Blanchard, E.B. (1988). Information and decision making preferences of hospitalised cancer patients. *Social Science and Medicine*, **27**, 1139–45.

Blanks, R.G., Given-Wilson, R.M., and Moss, S. (1998). Efficiency of cancer detection during routine repeat (incident) mammographic screening: two view versus one view mammography. *Journal of Medical Screening*, **5**, 141–5.

Blaxter, M. (1983). The causes of disease—women talking. *Social Science and Medicine*, **17**, 59–69.

Blum, D. and Blum, R. (1991). Patient-team communication. *Journal of Psycosocial Oncology*, **9**, 81–8.

Boccardo, F., Rubagotti, A., Amoroso, D. *et al.* (1992). Chemotherapy versus tamoxifen versus chemotherapy plus tamoxifen in node-positive, oestrogen-receptor positive breast cancer patients. An update at 7 years of the first GROCTA (Breast Cancer Adjuvant Chemo-hormone Therapy Group) trial. *European Journal of Cancer*, **28**, 673–80.

Bonadonna, G., Veronesi, U., Brambilla, C. *et al.* (1990). Primary chemotherapy to avoid mastectomy in tumours with diameters of three centimeters or more. *Journal of the National Cancer Institute*, **82**, 1539–45.

Bonadonna, G., Pinuccia, M. D., Valagussa, B. S. *et al.* (1995). Adjuvant cyclophosphamide, methotrexate and fluorouracil in node-positive breast cancer. The results of 20 years of follow-up. *New England Journal of Medicine*, **332**, 901–6.

Bond, S. and Thomas, L. (1992). Measuring patients' satisfaction with nursing care. *Journal of Advanced Nursing*, **17**, 52–63.

Bottomley, A. (1997) Breast cancer care: women's experience. *European Journal of Cancer Care*, **6**, 124–32.

Boudioni, M. and Mossman, J. CancerBACUP, unpublished data.

Bowling, A. (1991). *Measuring health*. Open University Press, Buckingham.

Brandt, B. (1991). Information needs and selected variables in patients receiving brachytherapy. *Oncology Nursing Forum*, **18**, 1221.

Brazier, J.E., Harper, R., Jones, N. M. B., O'Caithan, A., and Thomas, K.J. (1992). Validating the SF36 health survey questionnaire: new outcome measure for primary care. *British Medical Journal*, **305**, 160–4.

British Association of Surgical Oncology (1994). Guide-lines for surgeons on the management of symptomatic breast disease in the United Kingdom. BASO, 35–43 Lincoln's Inn fields, London.

British Breast Group (1994). (Report of a working party of Richards, M.A., Baum, M., Dowsett, M., Maguire, P., McPherson, K., Morgan,

D.A.L., Sainsbury, R., Sloane, J., Wilson, R., Blamey., R., and Leake, R.) Provision of breast care services in the UK: the advantages of specialist breast units. *The Breast,* 3 (suppl.), 2–20.

British Medical Association (1981). *Handbook of medical ethics.* British Medical Association, London.

Brody, D.S., Miller, S.M., Lerman, C.E., Smith, D.G., and Caputo, G. (1989). Patient perception of involvement in medical care. *Journal of General Internal Medicine,* 4, 506–11.

Brooking, J. (1989). A survey of current practices and opinions concerning patient and family participation in hospital care. In: J. Wilson-Barnett, J. Robinson (eds.), *Directions in Nursing Research,* pp. 97–106. Scutari Press, London.

Brown, S.R., Ross, B., Peck, R., Shorthouse, A.J., Nutton, S., and Reed, M.W.R. (1997). The difficult screening mammogram: value of early follow up. *The Breast,* 6, 214–16.

Buckman, R. (1986). *Communicating with the patient, in coping with cancer stress* (ed. B.A. Stoll), pp. 165–73. Martinus Nijhoff Publications, The Netherlands.

Buckman, R. (1992). *How to break bad news: a guide to health care professionals.* Macmillan, London.

Bull, A.R. and Campbell, M. J. (1991). Assessment of the psychological impact of a breast screening programme. *British Journal of Radiology,* 64, 510–15.

Burns, N. and Grove, S.K. (1987). *The practice of nursing research, conduct, critique and utilisation,* pp. 291–5. W. B Saunders and Co, Philadelphia.

Burton, L. (1975). *The family life of sick children.* Routledge and Kegan Paul, London.

Bush, T., Fried, L., and Barratt-Connor (1988). Cholesterol lipoproteins and coronary heart disease in women. *Clinical Chemistry,* 34, B60–70.

Calabresi, G. and Bobbit, P. (1978). *Tragic choices,* p. 196. Norton, New York.

Calman Report (1995). *A policy framework for commissioning cancer services, expert advisory group on cancer to the chief medical officer.* Department of Health, London.

Calvin, J. (1960a). *Institutes of the Christian Religion,* Book 1 (ed. J. T. McNeill). Westminster Press, Philadelphia.

Calvin, J. (1960b). *Institutes of the Christian Religion,* Book 2 (ed. J. T. McNeill). Westminster Press, Philadelphia.

Cancer Relief Macmillan Fund (1994). *Breast cancer. How to help yourself.* Cancer Relief Macmillan Fund.

Cancer Research Campaign (1996). *Breast cancer fact sheet* (6.1). Cancer Research Campaign, Oxford.

Cancer Research Campaign Working Party in Breast Conservation (1983). Informed consent: ethical legal, and medical implications for doctors and patients who participate in randomised clinical trials. Vol. **286**, 1117–21. Cancer Research Campaign, Oxford.

Canterbury v. Spence (1972). The 'Prudent Patient' standard, 464 F 2d, DC1972.

Cardozo, J. (1914). In *Schloendorff v. Society of New York Hospital*, 105 NE92, New York.

Cartwright, A. (1964). *Human relations and hospital care*. Routledge and Kegan Paul, London.

Cassileth, B.R., Zupkis, R.V., Sutton-Smith, K., and March, V. (1980). Information and participation preferences of hospitalised adult cancer patients. *Annals of Internal Medicine*, **92**, 832–6.

Chapman, G.B., Elstein, A.S., and Kostbade Huges, K. (1995). Effects of patient education on decisions about breast cancer treatments. *Medical Decision Making*, **15**, 231–9.

Charles, C., Redko, C., Whelan, T., Gafni, A., and Reyno, L. (1996). *Doing nothing is no choice: lay constructions of treatment decision-making among women with early stage breast cancer*. Hamilton McMaster University Centre for Health Economics and Policy Analysis. Working Paper 96–17.

Charles, C., Gafni, A., and Whelan, T. (1997). Shared decision-making in the medical encounter: What does it mean? (or it takes at least two to tango). *Social Science and Medicine*, **44**, 681–92.

Cimprich, B. (1993). Development of an intervention to restore attention in cancer patients. *Cancer Nursing*, **16**, 83–92.

Claus, E.B., Risch, N. and Thompson, W. D. (1990). Age at onset as an indicator of familial risk of breast cancer. *American Journal of Epidemiology*, **131**, 961–72.

Claus, E.B., Risch, N. and Thompson, W. D. (1991). Genetic analysis of breast cancer in the cancer and steroid hormone study. *American Journal of Human Genetics*, **48**, 232–42.

Clough, A.H. (1977). The latest decalogue. In *Causing death and saving lives* (ed. J. Glover), p. 92. Penguin, Harmondsworth.

Coates, A.S. and Simes, R.J. (1992). In *Introducing new treatments for cancer, practical, ethical and legal problems* (ed. C.J. Williams), pp. 447–58. John Wiley, London.

Cole, M.P., Jones, C.T.A., and Todd, I.D.H. (1971). A new antioestrogenic agent in late breast cancer. An early appraisal of ICI 46, 474. *British Journal of Cancer*, **25**, 270–5.

Cook, D. (1983). *The Moral Maze*. SPCK, London.

Cooley, M.E., Moriarty, H., Berger, M.S. *et al.* (1995). Patient literacy and the readability of written educational materials. *Oncology Nursing Forum*, **22**, 1345–50.

232   References

Copp, L.A. (1986). The nurse as advocate for vulnerable persons. *Journal of Advanced Nursing*, **11**, 255–63.
Costantino, J., Kuller, L., Ives, D. *et al.* (1997). Coronary heart disease mortality and adjuvant tamoxifen therapy. *Journal of the National Cancer Institute*, **89**, 776–82.
Cotton, T., Locker, A.P., Jackson, L., Blamey, R.W., and Morgan, D.A.L. (1991). A prospective study of patient choice in treatment for primary breast cancer. *European Journal of Surgical Oncology*, **17**, 115–7.
Cornwell, J. (1984). *Hard-earned lives: accounts of health and illness from East London*. Tavistock Publications, London.
Coulter, A. (1997). Partnerships with patients: the pros and cons of shared clinical decision-making. *Journal of Health Services Research and Policy*, **2**, 112–21.
Coulter, A., Entwistle, V., and Gilbert, D. (1998). *Informing patients: assessing the quality of patient information materials*. King's Fund, London.
Craufurd, D., Dodga, A., Kerzin-Storrar, L., and Harris, R. (1989). Uptake of presymptomatic predictive testing for Huntington's disease. *Lancet*, **ii**, 603–5.
Craufurd, D., Evans, D.G.R., and Binchy, A. (1995). *Response to BRCA1 (linkage) testing*. Poster presented to the Cancer Family Study Group, Manchester.
Current Trials Working Party of the Cancer Research Campaign Breast Cancer Trials Group (1996). Preliminary results from the Cancer Research Campaign trial evaluating tamoxifen duration in women aged fifty years or older with breast cancer. *Journal of the National Cancer Institute*, **88**, 1834–9.
Curtis, J. and Lacey, A. (1996). Measuring the quantity and quality of information-giving to in-patients. *Journal of Advanced Nursing*, **24**, 674–81.
Daily Mail (1997). March 11. pp. 103–5.
Dean, C., Chetty, U.and Forrest, A.P.M. (1983). Effects of immediate breast reconstruction on psychological morbidity after mastecomy. *Lancet*, **i**, 459–62.
Deardorff, W. (1986). Computerised health education, a comparison of traditional formats. *Health Education Quarterly* **13**, 61–72.
Deber, R.B. (1994). The patient-physician partnership: changing roles and the desire for information. *Canadian Medical Association Journal*, **151**, 171–6.
Deber, R. B. (1996). Editorial: Shared decision making in the real world. *Journal of General Internal Medicine*, **11**, 377–8.
Degner, L.F. and Aquino Russell, C.C.A. (1988). Preferences for treatment control among adults with cancer. *Res. Nursing Health*, **11**, 367–74.

Degner, L.F. and Sloane J.A. (1992). Decision-making during serious illness: what role do patients really want to play? *Journal of Clinical Epidemiology*, **45**, 941–50.

Degner, L.F., Kristjanson, L.J., Bowman, D., Sloan, J.A., Carriere, K.C., O'Neil, J., Bilodeau, B., Watson, P., and Mueller, B. (1997). Information needs and decisional preferences in women with breast cancer. *Journal of the American Medical Association*, **277**, 1485–92.

Department of Health (1990). *A guide to consent for examination or treatment*. HMSO, London.

Department of Health (1992). *The Patients' Charter*. HMSO, London.

Denton, S. (ed.), (1996). *Breast cancer nursing*. Chapman and Hall, London.

Early Breast Cancer Trialists' Collaborative Group (1992). Systemic treatment of early breast cancer by hormonal, cytotoxic or immune therapy. *Lancet*, **339**, 1–15, 71–85.

Early Breast Cancer Trialist's Collaborative Group (1995). Effects of radiotherapy and surgery in early breast cancer: an overview of the randomised trials. *New England Journal of Medicine*, **333**, 1444–5.

Early Breast Cancer Trialists' Collaborative Group (1996). Ovarian ablation in early breast cancer: overview of the randomised trials. *Lancet*, **348**, 1189–96.

Early Breast Cancer Trialists' Collaborative Group (1998). Tamoxifen for early breast cancer: an overview of the randomised trials. *Lancet*, **351**, 1451–67.

Easton, D.F. and Peto, J. (1990). The contribution of inherited predisposition to cancer incidence. *Cancer Surveys*, **9**, 395–415.

Easton, D.F., Bishop, D.T., Ford, D., Crockford, G.P., and the Breast Cancer Linkage Consortium (1993). Genetic linkage analysis in familial breast and ovarian cancer: results from 214 families. *American Journal of Human Genetics*, **52**, 678–701.

Easton, D.F., Ford, D., Bishop, D.T., and the Breast Cancer Linkage Consortium (1995). Breast and ovarian cancer incidence in *BRCA1* carriers. *American Journal of Human Genetics*, **56**, 265–71.

Eeles, R. A. (1993). Predictive testing for germline mutations in the *TP53* gene: are all the questions answered? *European Journal of Cancer*, **29**, 1361–5.

Ellis, D.A., Hopkin, J.M., Leitch, A.G., and Crofton, J. (1986). Doctor's orders: controlled trial of supplementary, written information for patients. *British Medical Journal*, I, 456.

Emanuel, E.J. and Emanuel, I.L. (1992). Four models of the physician-patient relationship. *Journal of the American Medical Association*, **267**, 2221–6.

Engelking, C. and Kalinowski, B.H. (1995). *A comprehensive guide to breast cancer treatment: current issues and controversies.* Triclinicia Communications, New York.

Evans, D.G.R., Maher, E.R., Maclead, R., Davies, D.R., Crauford, D. (1997). Uptake of genetic testing for cancer predisposition – ethical issues. *Journal of Medical Genetics,* 34, 746–9.

Evers-Kiebooms, G., Fryns, J.P., and Demyttenaere, K. (1996). Predictive and preimplantation genetic testing for Huntington's disease and other late onset dominant disorders: not in conflict but complementary. *Clinical Genetics,* 50, 275–6.

Evers-Kiebooms, G., Decruyenaere, M., Fryns, J.P., and Demyttenaere, K. (1997). Psychological consequences of presymptomatic testing for Huntington's disease. *Lancet,* 349, 808.

Fallowfield, L. (1997). Offering choice of surgical treatment to women with breast cancer. *Patient Education and Counseling,* 30, 209–14.

Fallowfield, L.J and Baum, M. (1989). Psychological welfare of patients with breast cancer. *Journal of the Royal Society of Medicine,* 82, 4–5.

Fallowfield, L.J., Baum, M., and Maguire, G.P. (1986). Effects of breast conservation on psychological morbidity associated with diagnosis and treatment of early breast cancer. *British Medical Journal,* 293, 1331–4.

Fallowfield, L.J., Baum, M., and Maguire, G.P. (1987). Addressing the psychological needs of the conservatively treated breast cancer patient: discussion paper. *Journal of the Royal Society of Medicine,* 80, 696–700.

Fallowfield, L.J., Hall, A., Maguire, G.P., and Baum, M. (1989). Does choice of treatment affect psychological morbidity in early breast cancer? A three year prospective study. *British Journal of Surgery,* 76, 641.

Fallowfield, L.J., Hall, A., Maguire, G.P., and Baum, M. (1990a). Psychological outcomes of different treatment policies in women with early breast cancer outside a clinical trial. *British Medical Journal,* 301, 575–80.

Fallowfield, L.J., Hall, A., Maguire, G.P., and Baum, M. (1990b). Psychological outcomes in women with early breast cancer. *British Medical Journal,* 301, 1394.

Fallowfield, L.J., Hall, A., Maguire, G.P., Baum, M., and A'Hern, R.P. (1994a). Psychological effects of being offered choice of surgery for breast cancer. *British Medical Journal,* 309, 448.

Fallowfield, L. J., Hall, A., Maguire, G. P., Baum, M., and A'Hern, R. P. (1994b). A question of choice: results of a prospective 3-year follow-up study of women with breast cancer, *The Breast,* 3, 202–8.

Faulder, C. (1985). 'Whose Body is it?'. In *The troubling issue of informed consent.* Virago Press, London.

Faulder, C. (1992). 'Better safe than sorry' Review. *Bulletin of Medical Ethics*, **75**, 29–33.

Feinmann, J. (1988). Consent on trial. *Nursing Times*, Nov. 2, **84**, 20.

Feldman, H.A., McKinlay, J.B., Potter, D.A., Freund, K.M., Burns, R. B., Moskowitz, M.A. *et al.* (1997). Nonmedical influences on medical decision making: an experimental technique using videotapes, factorial design, and survey sampling. *Health Services Research*, **32**, 343–66.

Fisher, B. and Anderson, S. (1994). Conservative surgery for the management of invasive and non-invasive carcinoma of the breast: NASBP Trials. *World Journal of Surgery*, **18**, 63–9.

Fisher, B., Constantino, J., Redmond, C. *et al.* (1994). Endometrial cancer in tamoxifen-treated breast cancer patients: findings from the National Surgical Adjuvant Breast and Bowel Project (NSABP) B-14. *Journal of the National Cancer Institute*, **86**, 527–37.

Fisher, B., Bauer, M., Margolese, R., Poisson, R., Pilch, Y., Redmond, C. *et al.* (1985). Five year results of a randomised clinical trial comparing total mastectomy and segmental mastectomy with or without radiation in the treatment of breast cancer. *New England Journal of Medicine*, **312**, 665–73.

Fisher, B., Constantino, J., Redmond, C. *et al.* (1989*a*). A randomised clinical trial evaluating tamoxifen in the treatment of patients with node-negative breast cancer who have estrogen-receptor-positive tumors. *New England Journal of Medicine*, **320**, 479–84.

Fisher, B., Redmond, C., Poisson, R., Margolese, R., Wolmark, N., Wickerham, L. *et al.* (1989*b*). Eight year results of a randomised clinical trial comparing total mastectomy and lumpectomy with or without irradiation in the treatment of breast cancer. *New England Journal of Medicine*, **320**, 822–8.

Fisher, B., Constantinao, J., Wickerham, L. *et al.* (1993). Adjuvant therapy for node-negative breast cancer: an update of the NSABP findings. *Proceedings of the American Society of Clinical Oncocology*, **12**, 69.

Fisher, B., Dignam, J., Bryant, J. *et al.* (1996). The worth of five versus more than five years of tamoxifen therapy for breast cancer patients with negative lymph nodes and estrogen receptor-positive tumours. *Journal of the National Cancer Institute*, **88**, 1529–42.

Fisher, L., Johnson, T., Porter, D., Bleich, H., and Slack, W. (1977). Collection of clean voided urine specimen: a comparison amongst spoken, written and computer based instructions. *American Journal of Public Health*, **67**, 640–4.

Fisher, V., Brown, A., Mamounas, E. *et al.* (1997). Effect of preoperative chemotherapy on local-regional disease in women with operable breast cancer: findings from National Surgical Adjuvant Breast and Bowel Project B-18. *Journal of Clinical Oncology*, **15**, 2483–93.

Fitzgerald, M.G., MacDonald, D., Krainer, M., Hoover, I., O'Neil, E., Unsal, H. *et al.* (1996). Germ-line mutations in Jewish and non-Jewish women with early-onset breast cancer. *New England Journal of Medicine*, **334**, 143–9.

Ford, D., Easton, D.F., Bishop, D.T., Narod, S.A., the Breast Cancer Linkage Consortium and Goldgar, D.E. (1994). Risks of cancer in *BRCA*1-mutation carriers. *Lancet*, **343**, 692–5.

Ford, D., Easton, D.F., and Peto, J. (1995). Estimates of the gene frequency of *BRCA*1 and its contribution to breast and ovarian cancer incidence. *American Journal of Human Genetics*, **57**, 1457–62.

Ford, D., Easton, D.F., Stratton, M.R., Narod, S., Goldgar, D., Derilee, P. *et al.* (1998). Genetic heterogeneity and penetrance analysis of the *BRCA*1 and *BRCA*2 genes in breast cancer families. *American Journal of Human Genetics*, **62**, 676–89.

Ford, S., Fallowfield, L., and Lewis, S. (1994). Can oncologists detect distress in their out-patients and how satisfied are they with their performance during bad news consultations? *British Journal of Cancer*, **70**, 767–70.

Fornander, T., Rutqvist, L.E., Cedermark, B. *et al.* (1989). Adjuvant tamoxifen in early breast cancer: occurrence of new primary cancers. *Lancet*, **i**, 117–20.

Forrest, A.P.M. (1986). *Breast cancer screening: report to the Health Ministers of England, Wales, Scotland and Northern Ireland*. HMSO, London.

Forrest, A.P., Stewart, H.J., Everington, D., Prescott, R.J., McArdle, C.S., Harnett, A. *et al.* (1996). Randomised controlled trial of conservation therapy for breast cancer: 6-year analysis of the Scottish trial. *Lancet*, **348**, 708–13.

France, E. (1998). BRCA1/2 mutation analysis: the hidden extras? Oral presentation to the Genetic Nurses Association Conference, London.

Franks, T.S., Manley, S., Thomas, A. *et al.* (1997). *BRCA1 and BRCA2 sequence analysis of 335 high-risk women*. Presented at the 47th Annual Meeting of the American Society of Human Genetics, Baltimore, USA.

Freudenheim, M. (1992). Software helps patients make crucial choices, *The New York Times*, Oct. 14, D6.

Gagliano, M.E. (1988). A literature review on the efficacy of video in patient education. *Journal of Medical Education*, **63**, 785–92.

Gail, M., Brintom, L., Byar, D. *et al.* (1989). Projecting individualised probabilities of developing breast cancer for white females who are examined annually. *Journal of the National Cancer Institute*, **81**, 1879–86.

Gantz, P.A. (1992). Treatment options for breast cancer—beyond survival. *New England. Journal of Medicine*, **326**, 1147.

Gayther, S.A., Warren , W., Mazoyer, S., Russell, P.A., Harrington, P.A., Chiano, M. *et al.* (1995). Germline mutations of the *BRCA1* gene in breast/ovarian cancer families: evidence for a genotype/phenotype correlation. *Nature Genetics*, **11**, 428–33.

Geisler, N.L. and Feinburg, P.D. (1980). *Introduction to Philosophy.* Baker Book House Company, Michigan.

Gillon, R. (1992). *Philosophical medical ethics*, pp. 60–6. John Wiley and Sons, Chichester.

Glover, J. (1990). *Causing death and saving lives.* Penguin, London.

Goldgar, D.E., Fields, P., Lewis, C.M., Tran, T.D., Cannon-Albright, L.A., Ward, J.H. *et al.* (1994). A large kindred with 17q-linked breast and ovarian cancer: genetic, phenotypic and geneological analysis. *Journal of the National Cancer Institute*, **86**, 200–9.

Goldie, L. (1982). The ethics of telling the patient. *Journal of Medical Ethics*, **8**, 128–33.

Gram, I.T., Lund, R., and Slenker, S. E. (1990). Quality of life following a false positive mammogram. *British Journal of Cancer*, **62**, 1018–22.

Gray, J. (1990). Psychological effects of breast cancer. *Nursing Standard*, March 4, pp. 27–9.

Graydon, J., Galloway, S., Palmer-Wickham, S., Harrison, D., Rich-van der Bij, L., West, P. *et al.* (1997). Information needs of women during early treatment for breast cancer. *Journal of Advanced Nursing*, **26**, 59–64.

Greer, S. (1979). Psychological response to breast cancer: effect on outcome. *Lancet*, **ii**, 785–7.

Greer, S. (1985). Cancer: psychiatric aspects. In *Recent advances in clinical psychology* (ed. K. Granville-Grossman), pp. 87–103. Churchill-Livingstone, London.

Greer, S. and Watson, M. (1987). Mental adjustment to cancer, its measurement and prognostic importance. *Cancer Surveys*, **6**, 439–53.

Greer, S., Morris, T., Pettingale, K.W., and Haybittle, J.L. (1990). Psychological response to breast cancer and 15 year outcome. *Lancet*, **335**, 49 f.

Griffiths, M. and Leek, C. (1995). Patient education needs: opinions of oncology nurses and their patients. *Oncology Nursing Forum*, **22**, 139–44.

Grogan, S., Conner, M., Willits, D., and Norman, P. (1995). Development of a questionnaire to measure patients' satisfaction with general practitioners' services. *British Journal of General Practice*, **45**, 525–9.

Gustafson, D.H., Wise, M., McTavish, F.M. *et al.* (1993). Development and pilot evaluation of a computer based support system for women with breast cancer. *Journal of Psychosocial Oncology*, **11**, 69–93.

Hack, T.F., Degner, L.F., and Dyck, D.G. (1994). Relationship between preferences for decisional control and illness information among women with breast cancer: a quantitative and qualitative analysis. *Social Science and Medicine*, **39**, 279–89.

Hakama, M., Holli, K., Isola, J., Kallioniemi, O. P., Karkkainen, A., Visakorpi, T. *et al.* (1995). Aggressiveness of screen-detected breast cancers. *Lancet*, **345**, 221–4.

Hall, J.M., Lee, M.K., Newman, B., Morrow, J.E., Anderson, L.A., Huey, B. *et al.* (1990). Linkage of early-onset familial breast cancer to chromosome 17q21. *Science*, **250**, 1684–9.

Han, X. and Liehr, J.G. (1992). Induction of covalent DNA adducts in rodents by tamoxifen. *Cancer Research*, **52**, 1360–3.

Hard, G., Iatropoulos, N., Jordan, K. *et al.* (1993). Major differences in the hepatocarcinogenicity and DNA adduct forming ability between toremifene and tamoxifen in female Crl: CD(BR) rats. *Cancer Research*, **53**, 4534–41.

Harris, J. (1985). *The value of life*, pp. 31–212. Routledge and Kegan Paul plc, London.

Harris, J.R., Morris, M., and Bonnadonna, G. (1993). Cancer of the breast. In *Cancer: principles and practice of oncology* (4th edn), (ed. V.T. DeVita Jr., S. Hellman, and S.A. Rosenberg), pp. 1246–332. JB Lippincott, Philadelphia.

Heidegger, M. (1962). *Being and time* (trans. J. Macquarrie and E. Robinson). Blackwell, Oxford.

Heyderman, E. (1996). *Coping with breast cancer*. Overcoming Common Problems series. Sheldon Press, London.

Hogbin, B. and Fallowfield, L. (1989). Getting it taped: the 'bad news' consultation with cancer patients. *British Journal of Hospital Medicine*, **41**, 330–2.

Holland, J.H. and Rowland, J.C. (1998). *Breast cancer handbook of psychooncology*. Oxford University Press, London.

Holt, J.T., Thompson, M.E., Szabo, C., Robinson-Benion, C., Arteaga, C.L., King, M.C. *et al.* (1996). Growth retardation and tumour inhibition by *BRCA1*. *Nature Genetics*, **12**, 298–302.

Hoskins, C.N. (1997). Breast cancer treatment-related patterns in side effects, psychological distress, and perceived health status. *Oncology Nursing Forum*, **24**, 1575–83.

Huggins, M., Bloch, M., Wiggins, S., Adam, S., Suchowersky, O., Trew, M. *et al.* (1992). Predictive testing for Huntington disease in Canada: adverse effects and unexpected results in those receiving a decreased risk. *American Journal of Medical Genetics*, **42**, 508–15.

Hughes, K.K. (1993). Decision making by patients with breast cancer: the role of information in treatment selection. *Oncology Nursing Forum*, **20**, 623–8.

Illanchazhian, S., Thangaraju, M., Sachdanandam, P. *et al.* (1995). Plasma lipids and lipoprotein alterations in tamoxifen-treated breast cancer women in relation to the menopausal status. *Cancer Biochemistry Biophysics*, **15**, 83–90.

Impicciatore, P., Pandolfini, C., Casella, N., and Bonati, M. (1997). Reliability of health information for the public on the world wide web: systematic survey of advice on managing fever in children at home. *British Medical Journal*, **314**, 1875–81.

Ingelfinger, F.J. (1980). Arrogance. *New England Journal of Medicine*, **303**, 1507–11.

Jacobson, J.A., Danforth, D.N., Cowan, K.H. *et al.* (1996). Ten year results of a comparison of conservation with mastectomy in treatment of stage I and II breast cancer, summary. *Evidence-Based Medicine*, **1**, 49.

Johnson, J.D., Roberts, C.S., Cox, C.E., Reintgen, D.S., Levine, J.S., and Parsons, M. (1996). Breast cancer patients' personality style, age, and treatment decision-making. *Journal of Surgical Oncology*, **63**, 183–6.

Jones, A., Powles, T., Treleaven, J., Burman, J., Nicolson, M., Chung, H.-I. *et al.* (1992). Haemostatic changes in thromboembolic risk during tamoxifen therapy in normal women. *British Journal of Cancer*, **66**, 744–7.

Jordan, V. (1976). Effect of tamoxifen (ICI 46,474) on initiation and growth of DMBA-induced rat mammary carcinomata. *European Journal of Cancer*, **12**, 419–25.

Jordan, V., Lababidi, M., and Mirecki, D. (1990). The antiestrogenic and antitumor properties of prolonged tamoxifen therapy in C3H/OUJ mice. *European Journal of Cancer*, **26**, 718–21.

Kant, I. (1964). Groundwork of the metaphysic of morals (1785). In *The moral law* (ed. H. J. Paton). Hutchinson University Library, London.

Kant, I. (1973). Critique of pure reason. In *Immanuel Kant's critique of pure reason* (ed. N. Kemp Smith). Macmillan, London.

Karp, S., Tonin, P., Begin, L. *et al.* (1997). Influence of BRCA1 mutations on nuclear grade and estrogen receptor status of breast carcinoma in Ashkenazi Jewish women. *Cancer*, **80**, 435–44

Kasper, J.F., Mulley, A.G., and Wennberg, J.E. (1992*a*). Developing shared decision-making programs to improve the quality of health care. *Journal of Quality Improvement*, **18**, 182–9.

Kasper, J.F., Mulley, A.G., and Wennberg, J.E. (1992*b*). Developing shared decision-making programs to improve the quality of health care. *Quality Review Bulletin*, **18**, 183–90.

Kedziera, P. and Levy, M.H. (1994). Collaborative practice in oncology. *Seminars in Oncology*, **21**, 705–11.

Kee, F. (1996). Patient's prerogatives and perceptions of benefit. *British Medical Journal*, **312**, 958–60.

Kennedy, I. (1988). The law and ethics of informed consent and randomised controlled trials. In *Treat me right*, pp. 213–24. Clarendon Press, Oxford.

Kerner, G.C. (1990). Three philosophical moralists. Clarendon Press, Oxford.

Kfir, N. (1989). *Crisis intervention verbatum*. Hemisphere, London.

Kfir, N. and Slevin, M. (1991). *From chaos to control, challenging cancer*, pp. 4–125. Tavistock and Routledge, London and New York.

Kings Fund Concensus Statement (1986). Treatment of early breast cancer. *British Medical Journal*, 293, 946–7.

Kings Fund Development Centre (1996). *Executive summary, the moral maze of practice*, pp. 1–6. Cavendish Square, London.

Kirby, J. (1983). Informed consent: what does it mean? *Journal of Medical Ethics*, 9, 69–75.

Klimowski, A. (1992). Kill or cure, how medicine exploits human drug tests. *Evening Standard*, Supplement, pp. 36–40.

Knowles, G. (1992). Helping cancer patients to retain information. *Nursing Times*, 88, 48 f.

Krishnasamy, M. (1996). What do cancer patients identify as supportive and unsupportive behaviour of nurses? A pilot study. *European Journal of Cancer Care*, 5, 103–10.

Kristensen, B., Ejiersten, B., Dalgaard, P. *et al.* (1994). Tamoxifen and bone metabolism in postmenopausal low-risk breast cancer patients: a randomised study. *Journal of Clinical Oncology*, 12, 992–7.

Laine, C. and Davidoff, F. (1996). Patient-centred medicine: a professional evolution. *Journal of the American Medical Association*, 275, 152–6.

Lalloo, F. *et al.* (1998). Fifth international psycho-oncology meeting in hereditary breast and ovarian cancer. Meeting abstract. Leuven.

Lancet (1998). Editorial. *The screening muddle. Lancet*, 351, 459.

Langston, A.A., Malone, K.E., Thompson, J.D., Daling, J.R. and Ostrander, E.A. (1996). *BRCA1* mutations in a population-based sample of young women with breast cancer. *New England Journal of Medicine*, 334, 137–42.

Laszweski, M. (1981). Patient advocacy in primary nursing. *Nursing Administration Quarterly*, 5, 28–30.

Legha, S. and Carter, S. (1976). Antiestrogens in the treatment of breast cancer. *Cancer Treatment Reviews*, 8, 205–16.

Legha, S., Buzdar, A., Hortobagyi, G. *et al.* (1979). Tamoxifen—use in treatment of metastatic breast cancer refractory to combination chemotherapy. *Journal of the American Medical Association*, 242, 49–52.

Lerman, C. E., Brody, D. S., Caputo, G. C., Smith, D. G., Lazaro, C. G., and Wolfson, H. G. (1990). Patients' perceived involvement in care scale: relationship to attitudes about illness and medical care. *Journal of General Internal Medicine*, 5, 29–33.

Lerman, C., Daly, M., Walsh, W. P., Resch, N., Seay, J., Barsevick, A. *et al.* (1993). Communication between patients with breast cancer and health care providers. Determinants and implications. *Cancer*, 72, 2616–20.

Lerman, C., Narod, S., Schulman, K., Hughes, C., Gomez-Caminero, A., Bonney, G. *et al.* (1996). BRCA1 testing in families with hereditary breast-ovarian cancer. A prospective study of patient decision making and outcomes. *Journal of the American Medical Association*, 275, 1885–92.

Levine, M. N., Gafni, A., Markham, B., and MacFarlane, D. (1992). A bedside instrument to elicit patients' preference concerning adjuvant chemotherapy for breast cancer. *Annals of Internal Medicine*, 117, 53–8.

Lewis, F. M. (1986). The impact of cancer on the family: a critical analysis of the research literature. *Patient Education and Counseling*, 269–89.

Ley, P. (1979). Memory and medical information. *British Journal of Social Clinical Psychology*, 8, 245–55.

Ley, P. (1988). *Communicating with patients: improving communication, satisfaction, and compliance*. Croom Helm, London.

Lippman, M. and Bolan, G. (1975). Oestrogen responsive human breast cancer in long-term tissue culture. *Nature*, 256, 592–3.

Lloyd, S., Watson, M., Waites, B., Meyer, L., Eeles, R., Ebbs, S. *et al.* (1996). Familial breast cancer: a controlled study of risk perception, psychological morbidity and health beliefs in women attending for genetic counselling. *British Journal of Cancer*, 74, 482–7.

Locker, D. and Dunt, D. (1978). Theoretical and methodological issues in sociological studies of consumer satisfaction and medical care. *Social Science and Medicine*, 12, 283–92.

Long, A. and Harrison, S. (1996). The balance of evidence. In *Evidence based decision making guide*, pp. 1–2. Health Service Journal.

Longman, A.J., Braden, C.J., and Mishel, M.H. (1997). Patterns of association over time of side-effects burden, self-help, and self-care in women with breast cancer. *Oncology Nursing Forum*, 24, 1555–60.

Love, R., Mazess, R., Barden, H., Epstein, S., Newcomb, P., Jordan, V. *et al.* (1992). Effects of tamoxifen on bone mineral density in postmenopausal women with breast cancer. *New England Journal of Medicine*, 326, 852–6.

Love, R., Wiebe, D., Feyzi, J. *et al.* (1994). Effects of tamoxifen on cardiovascular risk factors in postmenopausal women after 5 years of treatment. *Journal of the National Cancer Institute*, 86, 1534–9.

Luker, K. and Caress, A. (1989). Rethinking patient education. *Journal of Advanced Nursing*, **14**, 711–18.

Luker, K., Leinster, S., Owens, G., Beaver, K., and Degner, I. (1993). *Preferences for information and decision making in women newly diagnosed with breast cancer: final report*. Research and Development Unit, University of Liverpool Department of Nursing, Liverpool.

Luker, K., Beaver, K., Leinster, S., Owens, G., Degner, I., and Sloane, J. A. (1995). The information needs of women newly diagnosed with breast cancer. *Journal of Advanced Nursing*, **22**, 134–41.

Lynch, H.T., Watson, P., Conway, T.A., Lynch, J.F., Slominski-Caster, S.M., Narod, S.A. *et al.* (1993). DNA screening for breast/ovarian cancer susceptibility based on linked markers. A family study. *Archives of Internal Medicine*, **153**, 1979–87.

McDonald, C., Alexander, F., Whyte, B. *et al.* (1995). Cardiac and vascular morbidity in women receiving adjuvant tamoxifen for breast cancer in a randomised trial. *The Scottish Cancer Trials Breast Group*, **311**, 977–80.

McGuire, D.B. (1979). Impact of hereditary melanoma on families. *Cancer Nursing*, **7**, 451–9.

McHorney, C.A., Ware, J.E., Rogers, W., Raczek, A.E., and Lu, J.F.R. (1992). The validity and relative precision of MOS short and long form health status scales and Dartmouth COOP charts: results from medical outcomes study. *Medical Care*, **30** (suppl.), 253–65.

McHorney, C.A., Ware, J.E., and Raczek, A.E. (1993). The MOS short form health survey; II Psychometric and clinical tests of validity in measuring physical and mental health constructs. *Medical Care*, **31**, 247–63.

McIlwaine, G. (1993). Satisfaction with the NHS breast screening programme: women's views. In *Breast screening acceptability, research and practice* (ed. J. Austoker and J. Patnick), pp. 14–16. NHSBSP Publication No. 28.

McKinlay, J.B., Burns, R.B., Durante, R., Feldman, H.A., Freund, K.M., Harrow, B.S. *et al.* (1997). Patient, physician and presentational influences on clinical decision making for breast cancer: results from a factorial experiment. *Journal of Evaluation in Clinical Practice*, **3**, 23–57.

McNeil, B.J., Parker, S.G., Sox, H.C., and Tversky, A. (1982). On the elicitation of preferences for alternative therapies. *New England Journal of Medicine*, **307**, 1259–62.

McTavish, F.M., Gustafson, D.H., Owens, B.H. *et al.* 1993. CHESS an inteactive computer system for women with breast cancer piloted with an underserved population. *Journal of the American Medical Association*, suppl. 599.

MacIntyre, A. (1980). *A short history of ethics*. Routledge and Kegan Paul Ltd, London.

MacDonald, M. (1990). Natural rights. In *Theories of rights* (ed. J. Waldron), pp. 21–40. Oxford University Press, New York.

Macleod C. (1982). Nurse-patient communication—an analysis of conversations from surgical wards. (ed. J. Wilson Barnett) Ten studies in patient care. *Nursing Research*.

Maguire, G.P. (1976). The psychological and social sequelae of mastectomy. In *Modern perspectives in the psychiatric aspects of surgery* (ed. J. Howells). Churchill-Livingstone, Edinburgh.

Maguire, G.P., Goldberg , D.P., Hobson, R.J., Margison, F., Moss, S., and O'Dowd, T. (1984). Evaluating the teaching of a method of psychotherapy. *British Journal of Psychotherapy*, **144**, 575–80.

Maguire, P.J. (1985). Barriers to psychological care of the dying. *British Medical Journal*, **291**, 1711–3.

Maguire, P.J. (1988). The psychological impact of cancer. *British Journal of Hospital Medicine*, **34**, 100–3.

Maguire, P.J. (1990). Can communication skills be taught? *British Journal of Hospital Medicine*, **43**, 215–16.

Maguire, P. and Faulkner, A. (1988*a*). Improve the counselling skills of doctors and nurses in cancer care. *British Medical Journal*, **297**, 847–9.

Maguire, P. and Faulkner, A. (1988*b*). Communicate with cancer patients: 1. Handling bad news and difficult questions. *British Medical Journal*, **297**, 907–9.

Maguire, P. and Faulkner, A. (1988*c*). Communicate with cancer patients: handling uncertainty, collusion, and denial. *British Medical Journal*, **297**, 972–4.

Maguire, P.J., Roe, P., and Goldberg, D. (1978). The value of feedback in teaching interviewing skills to medical students. *Psychological Medicine*, **8**, 695–704.

Maguire, P.J., Tait, A., Brook, M., Thomas, C., and Sellwood, R. (1980). Effect of counselling on the psychiatric morbidity associated with mastectomy. *British Medical Journal*, **281**,1454–6.

Maguire, P.J., Pentol, A., Allen, D. *et al.* (1982). The cost of counselling women who undergo mastectomy. *British Medical Journal*, **284**, 1933–5.

Maguire, P.J., Brook, M., Tait, A. *et al.* (1983). The effect of counselling on physical disability and social recovery after mastectomy. The psychiatric morbidity associated with mastectomy. *Clinical Oncology*, **9**, 319–24.

Maguire, P.J., Faribairn, S., and Fletcher, C. (1986). Consultation skills of young doctors. *British Medical Journal*, **292**, 1573–6.

Mahon, S.M. and Caspeson, D.S. (1995). Hereditary cancer syndrome: Part 2 Psychosocial issues, concerns and screening—results of a qualitative study. *Oncology Nurses Forum*, 22, 775–82.

Majeed, A.F., Cook, D.G., Given-Wilson, R.M., Vecchi, P., and Poloniecki, J. (1995). Do general practitioners influence the uptake of breast cancer screening? *Journal of Medical Screening*, 2, 119–24.

Manni, A., Trujillo, J., Marshall, J. *et al.* (1976). Antiestrogen-induced remissions of stage IV breast cancer. *Cancer Treatment Reports*, 60, 1145–50.

Marteau, T.M., Kidd, J., Cook, R., Michie, S., Johnston, M., Slack, J. *et al.* (1991). Perceived risk not actual risk predicts uptake of amnoicentesis. *British Journal of Obstetrics and Gynaecology*, 98, 282–6.

Maslin, A.M. (1993). A survey of the opinions of women in a breast unit on the issues of giving consent to joining a clinical trial. Unpublished MSc. Thesis, University of Surrey Library, Guildford, England.

Maslin, A. M. (1994). A survey of the opinions on 'informed consent' of women currently involved in clinical trials within a breast unit. *European Journal of Cancer Care*, 3, 153–62.

Maslin, A.M., Powles, T.J., Baum, M., Ashley, S., and Tidy, V.A. (1993). A survey of the opinions on informed consent of women attending a breast unit. *The Breast*, 2, 208.

Maslin, A.M., Baum, M., Secker Walker, J., A'Hern, R., and Prouse, A. (1998). Shared decision making using an interactive video disk system for women with early breast cancer. *Nursing Times*, 3, 444–54.

Meade, C.D., McKinney, P., and Barnas, G.P. (1994). Educating patients with limited literacy skills: the effectiveness of printed and videotaped materials about colon cancer. *American Journal of Public Health*, 84, 119–21.

Medical Research Council (1962/3). Report of responsibilities in investigations on human subjects. HMSO 2382, London.

Melia, K. (1985). Informed consent, dangerous territory. *Nursing Times*, May 21, p. 27.

Meredith, C., Symonds, P., Webster, L., Lamont, D., Pyper, E., Cillis, C.R. *et al.* (1996). Informational needs of cancer patients in west Scotland: cross sectional survey of patients' views. *British Medical Journal*, 313, 724–6.

Meyer, B.J.F., Russo, C., and Talbot, A. (1995). Discourse comprehension and problem solving: decisions about the treatment of breast cancer by women across the life span. *Psychology and Aging*, 10, 84–103.

Miki, Y., Swensen, J., Shattuck-Eidens, D., Futreal, P.A., Harshman, K., Tavtigian, S. *et al.* (1994). A strong candidate for the breast and ovarian cancer susceptibility gene, BRCA1. *Science*, 266, 66–71.

Mill, J.S. (1962a). Utilitarianism 1861. In *Utilitarianism* (ed. M. Warnock), p. 289. William Collins, Glasgow.

Mill, J.S. (1962*b*). On liberty 1859. In *Utilitarianism* (ed. M. Warnock). Collins/Fontana, London.

Mill, J.S. (1974). Utilitarianism. In *Utilitarianism* (ed. M. Warnock), p. 268. Fontana, Glasgow.

Miller, W.R., Ellis, I.O., and Sainsbury, J.R.C. (1995). Prognostic factors. In *ABC of breast diseases* (ed. J. M. Dixon). BMJ Publishing group.

Mitretek Systems (1997). Criteria for assessing the quality of health information on the internet. http://www.mitretek.org

Morales, M., Sanana, N., Soria, A. *et al.* (1996). Effects of tamoxifen on serum lipid and apolipoprotein levels in postmenopausal patients with breast cancer. *Breast Cancer Research and Treatment*, 40, 265–70.

Moran, N. (1995). Treatment choices from evidence based medicine. *Nature Medicine*, 1, 1114–15.

Morris, J. and Ingham, R. (1988). Choice of surgery for breast cancer: psychosocial considerations. *Social Science and Medicine*, 27, 1257–62.

Morris, J. and Royle, G. (1988). Offering patients a choice of surgery for early breast cancer: a reduction in anxiety and depression in patients and their husbands. *Social Science and Medicine*, 26, 583–5.

Morris, T. (1983). Psychological aspects of breast cancer; a review. *European Journal of Clinical Oncology*, 19, 1725–33.

Mort, E.A. (1996). Clinical decision-making in the face of scientific uncertainty: HRT as an example. *The Journal of Family Practice*, 42, 147–51.

Mort, E.A., Esserman, L., Tripathy, D., Hillner, B., Houghton, J., Bunker, J.P. *et al.* (1995). Diagnosis and management of early stage breast cancer. *JCOM: Obstetrics and Gynaecology*, 1, 1–16.

Mulley, A.G. (1990). Supporting the patient's role in clinical decision making. *Journal of Occupational Medicine*, 32, 1227–8.

Mulley, A. G. (1992). The patient's role in clinical decision making. *Cardiology*, 2, 8.

Mulley, A.G. (1994). Outcome research: implications for policy and practice. In *Outcome into clinical practice* (ed. T. Delamoth), pp. 13–27. BMJ Publishing Group, London.

Narod, S.A., Feunteun, J., Lynch, H.T., Watson, P., Conway, T., Lynch, J. *et al.* (1991). Familial breast-ovarian cancer locus on chromosome 17q12-q23. *Lancet*, 338, 82–3.

Nayfield, S. and Gorling, M. (1996). Tamoxifen-associated eye disease. A review. *Journal of Clinical Oncology*, 14, 1018–26.

Naylor, C.D. (1995). Grey zones of clinical practice: some limits to evidence-based medicine. *Lancet*, 345, 840–2.

Neilsen, E. and Sheppard, M.A. (1988). Television as a patient education tool: a review of its effectiveness. *Patient Education Counselling*, 11, 3–16.

Nelkin, D. (1992). The social power of genetic information. In *The code of codes* (ed. D.J. Kevles and L. Hood), pp. 177–90. Harvard University Press, Cambridge, Massachusetts.

Neuhausen, S., Gilewski, T., Norton, L., Tran, T., McGuire, P., Swensen, J. *et al.* (1996). Recurrent BRCA2 6174delT mutations in Ashkenazi Jewish women affected by breast cancer. *Nature Genetics*, **13**, 126–8.

NHS Executive, Cancer Guidance Sub-group of the Clinical Outcomes Group (1996). *Guidance for purchasers, improving outcomes in breast cancer, the manual.*

NHS Executive, Cancer Guidance Sub-group of the Clinical Outcomes Group (1996). *Guidance for purchasers, improving outcomes in breast cancer, the research evidence.*

Northouse, L. (1988). The impact of cancer on the family: an overview. *International Journal of Psychiatry Medicine*, **14**, 215–43.

Oberst, M.T., Chang, A.S., and McCubbin, M.A. (1991). Self-care burden, stress appraisal, and mood among persons receiving radiotherapy. *Cancer Nursing*, **14**, 71–8.

Oddoux, C., Struewing, J.P., Clayton, C.M., Neuhausen, S., Brody, L.C., Kaback, M. *et al.* (1996). The carrier frequency of the BRCA2 6174delT mutation among Ashkenazi Jewish individuals is approximately 1%. *Nature Genetics*, **14**, 188–90.

Offit, K., Gilewski, T., McGuire, P., Schluger, A., Hampel, H., Brown, K. *et al.* (1996). Germline BRCA1 185delAG mutations in Jewish women with breast cancer. *Lancet*, **347**, 1643–5.

Ong, G. and Austoker, J. (1997). Recalling women for further investigation of breast screening: women's experiences at the clinic and afterwards. *Journal of Public Health Medicine*, **19**, 29–36.

Overgaard, M., Hansen, P.S., Overgaard, J., Rose, C., Andersson, M., Bach, F. *et al.* (1997). Postoperative radiotherapy in high-risk premenopausal women with breast cancer who receive adjuvant chemotherapy. *New England Journal of Medicine*, **337**, 949–55.

Palsson, M.-B.E. and Norberg, A. (1995). Breast cancer patients' experiences of nursing care with the focus on emotional support: the implementation of a nursing intervention. *Journal of Advanced Nursing*, **21**, 277–85.

Palvidis, N., Petris, C., Briassoulis, E. *et al.*, (1992). Clear evidence that long term, low dose tamoxifen treatment can induce ocular toxicity. A prospective study of 63 patients. *Cancer*, **69**, 2961–4.

Parkin, D. (1976). Survey of the success of communications between hospital staff and patients. *Public Health*, **90**, 203–9.

Pathak, D. and Bodell, W. (1994). DNA adduct formation by tamoxifen with rat and human liver microsomal activation systems. *Carcinogenesis*, **15**, 529–32.

The Patients' Charter (1992, 1995). Department of Health, HMSO, London.

Patnick, J. (ed.), (1996). *NHS breast screening programme review 1996.* NHS Breast Screening Programme.

Powles, T.J., Hickish, T.F., Makris, A., Ashley, S.E., O'Brien, M.E.R., Tidy, V.A. *et al.* (1995). Randomised trial of chemoendocrine therapy started before or after surgery for treatment of primary breast cancer. *Journal of Clinical Oncology*, 13, 547–52.

Powles, T. J and Hickish, T. (1995). Tamoxifen therapy and carcinogenic risk. Editorial. *Journal of the National Cancer Institute*, 87, 1343–4.

Powles, T.J. and Smith, I.E. (1991). *Medical management of breast cancer.* Martin Duntitz Ltd, London. Cambridge University Press.

Powles, T., Tillyer, C., Jones, A., Ashley, S., Treleaven, J., Davey, J. *et al.* (1990). Prevention of breast cancer with tamoxifen—an update on the Royal Marsden Hospital pilot programme. *European Journal of Cancer*, 26, 680–4.

Powles, T.J., Jones, A.L., Ashley, S.E., O'Brien, M.E.R., Tidy, V.A., Casey, S. *et al.* (1994). The Royal Marsden Hospital pilot tamoxifen chemoprevention trial. *Breast Cancer Research Treatment*, 31, 73–82.

Powles, T.J., Hickish, T., Kanis, J.A., Tidy, A., and Ashley, S. (1996). Effect of tamoxifen on bone mineral density measured by dual-energy X-ray absorptiometry in healthy premenopausal and postmenopausal women. *Journal of Clinical Oncology*, 14, 78–84.

Priestman, T.J. (1986). Impact of diagnosis on the patient. In *Coping with cancer stress* (ed. B.A. Stoll), pp. 22–7. Martinus Nijhoff Publications, The Netherlands.

Pyne, R. (1986). Tell Me Honestly. *Nursing Times*, May 21, pp. 25–6.

Quill, T.E. (1983). Partnerships in patient care: a contractual approach. *Annals of Internal Medicine*, 98, 228–34.

Ragaz, J., Jackson, S.M., Le, N., Plenderleith, I.H., Spinelli, J.J., Basco, V.E. *et al.* (1997). Adjuvant radiotherapy and chemotherapy in node-positive pre-menopausal women with breast cancer. *New England Journal of Medicine*, 337, 956–62.

Rapheal, W. (1969). *Patients and their hospitals.* King Edwards Hospital Fund, London.

Rawlings, G. (1992). Ethics and regulation in randomised controlled trials of therapy. In *Challenges in medical care* (ed. A. Grubb), pp. 29–58. John Wiley and Sons, New York.

Read, C. (1995). *Preventing breast cancer, the politics of an epidemic.* Harper Collins, London.

Ream, E. and Richardson, A. (1996). The role of information in patients' adaptation to chemotherapy and radiotherapy: a review of the literature. *European Journal of Cancer Care*, 5, 132–8.

Redmond, C. and Costantino, J. (1996). Design and current status of the NSABP breast cancer prevention trial (BCPT). Proceedings of adjuvant therapy of cancer. *Recent Results in Cancer Research*, **140**, 309–17.

Reynolds, M. (1978). No news is bad news: patients views about communication in hospital. *British Medical Journal*, **1**, 1673–6.

Reynolds, S.A., Sachs, S.H., Davis, J.M., and Hall, P. (1981). Meeting the information needs of patients on clinical trials a new approach. *Cancer Nursing*, June, 227–30.

Ribeiro, G. and Swindell, R. (1992). The Christie Hospital adjuvant tamoxifen trial. *Monographs of the National Cancer Institute*, **11**, 121–5.

Richards, M.A., Ramirez, A.J., Degner, L.F., Fallowfield, L.J., Maher, E.J., and Neuberger, J. (1995). Offering choice of treatment to patients with cancer. *European Journal of Cancer*, **31A**, 112–16.

Richards, M.P.M. (1996). Lay and professional knowledge of genetics and inheritance. *Public Understanding Science*, **5**, 217–30.

Rijken, M., Anja de Kruif, A.T., Komproe, I.H., and Roussel, J.G. (1995). Depressive symptomatology of post-menopausal breast cancer patients: a comparison of women recently treated by mastectomy or by breast-conserving therapy. *European Journal of Surgical Oncology*, **21**, 498–503.

Roa, B.B., Boyd, A.A., Volcik, K. and Richards, C.S. (1996). Ashkenazi Jewish population frequencies for common mutations in BRCA1 and BRCA2. *Nature Genetics*, **14**, 185–7.

Roberts, M. (1989). Critique of the mammography screening service. *British Medical Journal*, **229**, 1153–5.

Roberts, R. (1990). Who supports the cancer counsellors? *Nursing Times*, Sept. 5, 32–4.

Roberts, R., and Fallowfield, L. (1990). The goals of cancer counsellors. *Counselling* **1**, 88–91.

Robinson, S., Langan-Fahey, L., Johnson, D., and Jordan, V. (1991). Metabolites, pharmacodynamics and pharmacokinetics of tamoxifen in rats and mice compared to the breast cancer patient. *Drug Metabolism Disposal*, **19**, 36–43.

Roper, W.L., Winkenwerder, W., Hackbarth, J.D., and Krakauer, H. (1988). Effectiveness in health care. *The New England Journal of Medicine*, **319**, 1197–202.

Ross, W.D. (1930). *The right and the good*. Oxford University Press, Oxford.

Rothert, M., Padonu, G., Holmes-Rovener, M., Kroll, J. *et al.* (1994). Menopausal women as decision makers in health care. *Experimental Gerontology*, **29**, 463–8.

Rowland, J.H. (1989). Intrapersonal resources: coping. In *Handbook of psychooncology* (ed. J.C. Holland and J.H. Rowland). Oxford University Press, New York.

Royal College of Nursing (1977). *Ethics related to research in nursing*, pp. 2–7. Royal College of Nursing.

Royal College of Nursing (1994). *Breast care nursing society standards of nursing care*. Royal College of Nursing.

Royal College of Physicians (1986). *Research on healthy volunteers, a working party*, pp. 3–17. Royal College of Physicians, London.

Royal College of Physicians (1990a). *Guide-lines on the practice of ethics committees in medical research involving human subjects, a working party*, pp. 20–5. Royal College of Physicians, London.

Royal College of Physicians (1990b) *Research involving patients, a working party*, pp. 3, 15–19, 42. Royal College of Physicians, London.

Rubens, R.D. (1992). Management of early breast cancer. *British Medical Journal*, **304**, 1361–4.

Rutqvist, L., Cedermark, B., Glas, U. *et al.* (1991). Contralateral primary tumours in breast cancer patients in a randomised trial of adjuvant tamoxifen therapy. *Journal of the National Cancer Institute*, **83**, 1299–1306.

Rutqvist, L., Johansson, H., Signomklao, T., Johansson, U., Fornander, T., and Wilking, N. (1995). Adjuvant tamoxifen therapy for early stage breast cancer and second primary malignancies. Stockholm Breast Cancer Study Group. *Journal of the National Cancer Institute*, **87**, 645–51.

Rutqvist, L.E., Liedberg, A., Hammar, N., and Dalberg, K. (1998). Myocardial infarction among women with early-stage breast cancer treated with conservative surgery and breast irradiation. *International Journal of Radiation Oncology*, **40**, 359–63.

Sacks, N.P.M. and Baum, M. (1993). Primary management of carcinomas of the breast. *Lancet,* **342**, 1402–7.

Saunders, C. and Baum, M. (1993). What is consent? Guide-lines in relation to consent and clinical research. *Surgery*. The Medicine Group (Journalists) Ltd.

Saunders, C.M. and Baum, M. (1994). Management of early breast cancer, oncology in practice. Ciba and European School of Oncology.

Saunders, C.M., Baum, M., and Houghton, J. (1994). Consent, research and the doctor-patient relationship. In *Principles of health care ethics* (ed. R. Gillon), pp. 457–69. John Wiley and Sons Ltd.

Scanlon, T.M. (1990). Rights, goals, and fairness. In *Theories of rights* (ed. J. Waldron), pp. 137–52. Oxford University Press, New York.

Schafer, A. (1989). Achieving informed consent in clinical trials. In *Ethical dilemmas in cancer care* (ed. B.A. Stoll), pp. 29–37. MacMillan Press, London.

Shapiro, D., Boggs, S., Melamed, B., and Graham-Pole, J. (1992). The effect of varied physician affect on recall, anxiety, and perceptions in women at risk of breast cancer: an analogue study. *Health Psychology*, **11**, 61–6.

Shattuck-Eidens, D., McClure, M., Simard, J., Labrie, F., Narod, S., Couch, F. *et al.* (1995). A collaborative survey of 80 mutations in the BRCA1 breast and ovarian cancer susceptibility gene. *Journal of the American Medical Association*, **273**, 535–41.

Shattuck-Eidens, D., Oliphant, A., McClure, M., McBride, C., Gupte, J., Rubano, T. *et al.* (1997). BRCA1 sequence analysis in women at high risk for susceptibility mutations. *Journal of the American Medical Association*, **278**, 1242–50.

Shepherd, S., Coulter, A., and Farmer, A. (1995). Using interactive videos in general practice to inform patients about treatment choices: a pilot study. *Family Practice*, **12**, 443–7.

Sidgwick, H. (1907). *The methods of ethics* (7th edn), Book 4, London.

Silverman, W. and Altman, D. (1996). Patient's preferences and randomised trials, *Lancet*, **347**, 171–4.

Siminoff, L.A., Fetting, J.H., and Abeloff, M.D. (1989). Doctor–patient communication about breast cancer adjuvent therapy. *Journal of Clinical Oncology*, **7**, 1192–200.

Simpson, M., Buckman, R., Stewart, M., Maguire, P., Lipkin, M., Novack, D. *et al.* (1991). Doctor–patient communication: the Toronto consensus statement. *British Medical Journal*, **303**, 1385–7.

Singer, P. (1994). *Ethics*. Oxford University Press, Oxford.

Slevin, M.L., Plant, H., Lynch, D. *et al.* (1988). Who should measure quality of life, the doctor or the patient? *British Journal of Cancer*, **57**, 109–12.

Slevin, M., Stubbs, L., Plant, H., Wilson, P., Gregory, W., Armes, P. *et al.* (1990). Attitudes to chemotherapy: comparing views of patients with cancer to those of doctors, nurses and general public. *British Medical Journal*, **300**, 1458–60.

Smith, I.E., Walsh, G., Jones, A. *et al.* (1995). High complete remission rates with primary neoadjuvant infusional chemotherapy for large early breast cancer. *Journal of Clinical Oncology*, **13**, 424–9.

Smitt, M.C. and Heltzel, M. (1997). Women's use of resources in decision-making for early-stage breast cancer: results of a community-based survey. *Annals of Surgical Oncology*, **4**, 564–9.

Sontag, S. (1991). *Illness as metaphor and aids and its metaphors*. Penguin, London.

Stewart, H., for the Scottish Cancer Trials Breast Group. The Scottish trial of adjuvant tamoxifen in node-negative breast cancer. *Monographs of the National Cancer Institute*, **11**, 117–20.

Stewart, H.J., Forrest, A.P., Everington, D. *et al.* (1996). Randomised comparison of 5 years of adjuvant tamoxifen with continuous therapy for operable breast cancer. The Scottish Cancer Trials Breast Group. *British Journal of Cancer*, **74**, 297–9.

Stewart, M.A. (1995). Effective physician-patient communication and health outcomes: a review. *Canadian Medical Association Journal*, **152**, 1423–33.

Street, R.L., Voigt, B., Geyer, C., Manning, T., and Swanson, G.P. (1995). Increasing patient involvement in choosing treatment for early breast cancer. *Cancer*, **76**, 2275–85.

Struewing, J.P., Abeliovich, D., Peretz, T., Avishai, N., Kaback, M.M., Collins, F.S. *et al.* (1995a). The carrier frequency of the *BCRA1* 185delAG mutation is approximately 1 per cent in Ashkenazi Jewish individuals. *Nature Genetics*, **11**, 198–200.

Struewing, J.P., Lerman, C., Kase, R.G., Giambarresi, T.R., Tucker, M.A. *et al.* (1995b). Anticipated uptake and impact of genetic testing in hereditary breast and ovarian cancer families. *Cancer Epidemiology Biomarkers Prevention*, **4**, 169–73.

Strull, M., Bernard, L., and Gerald, C. (1984). Do patients want to participate in medical decision making? *Journal of the American Medical Association*, **252**, 2990–4.

Suominen, T. (1992). Breast cancer patients' opportunities to participate in their care. *Cancer Nursing*, **15**, 68–72.

Suominen, T. (1993). How do nurses assess the information received by breast cancer patients? *Journal of Advanced Nursing*, **18**, 64–8.

Sutherland, H.J., Llewellyn-Thomas, H.A., Lockwood, G.A., Trichler, D.L. and Till, J.E. (1989). Cancer patients, their desire for information and participation in treatment decisions. *Journal of the Royal Society of Medicine*, **82**, 260–3.

Swedish Breast Cancer Cooperative Group (1996). Randomised trial of two versus five years of adjuvant tamoxifen for postmenopausal early stage breast cancer. *Journal of the National Cancer Institute*, **88**, 1543–9.

Szasz, T.S. and Hollender, M.H. (1956). A contribution to the philosophy of medicine. *Archives of Internal Medicine*, **97**, 585–92.

Tabar, L., Fagerberg, G., Day, N.E., Duffy, S.W., and Kitchin, R.M. (1992). Breast cancer treatment and natural history: new insights from results of screening. *Lancet*, **339**, 412–14.

Tang, R., Shjields, J., Schiffman, J. *et al.* (1997). Retinal changes associated with tamoxifen treatment for breast cancer. *Eye*, **11**, 295–7.

Thangaraju, M., Kumar, K. Gandhirajan, R. *et al.* (1994). Effect of tamoxifen on plasma lipids and lipoproteins in postmenopausal women with breast cancer. *Cancer*, **73**, 659–63.

Thomas, S., Glynne-Jones, R., and Chait, I. (1997). Is it worth the wait? A survey of patients' satisfaction with an oncology outpatient clinic. *European Journal of Cancer Care*, 6, 50–8.

Thornton, H.M. (1992). Breast cancer trials: a patient's viewpoint. *Lancet*, 339, 44–5.

Tibben, A., Vegter van der Vis, M., Niermeijer, M.E., Kamp, J.J., Roos, R.A., Rooijmans, H.G. *et al.* (1990). Testing for Huntington's disease with support for all parties. *Lancet*, 335, 553.

Tobias, J.S. (1988). Informed consent and controlled trials. *Lancet*, Nov. 19, 1194.

Tongue, B. (1991). A video based system for patients. *Health Trends*, 23, 11–12.

Tonin, P., Weber, B., Offit, K., Couch, F., Rebbeck, T.R., Neuhausen, S. *et al.* (1996). A high frequency of *BRCA1* and *BRCA2* mutations in 222 Ashkenazi Jewish breast cancer families. *Nature Medicine*, 2, 1179–83.

Tournier, P. (1957). *The meaning of persons*. SCM Press Ltd, London.

Tyron, P.A. and Leonard, R. C. (1965). Giving the patient an active role. In *Social interaction and patient care* (ed. J. K. Skipper and R.C. Leonard). Lippincott, Philadelphia.

UKCC (1989). *Exercising Accountability* (2nd edn), pp. 12–3. United Kingdom Central Council for Nursing, Midwifery and Health Visiting, London.

de Vahl Davis, V. (1992). How informed is informed consent? *Bulletin of Medical Ethics*, March, No. 76.

Valanis, G. and Rumpler C.H. (1985). Helping women to choose breast cancer treatment alternatives. *Cancer Nursing*, 8, 167–75.

Veatch, R.M. (1972). Models for ethical medicine in a revolutionary age: what physician-patient roles foster the most ethical relationship? *Hastings Center Report*, 2, 5–7.

Verhoog, L.C., Brekelmans, C.T.M., Seynaeve, C., Van den Bosch, L.M.C., Dahmen, G., Van Geel, A.N. *et al.* (1998). Survival and tumour characteristics of breast cancer patients with germline mutations of BRCA1. *Lancet*, 351, 316–21.

Wagener, J.J. and Taylor, S.E. (1986). What else could I have done? Patients' responses to failed treatment options. *Health Psychology*, 5, 481–96.

Wagner, E., Barrett, P., Barry, M., Barlow, W., and Fowler, F. (1993). The effect of a shared decision making programme on rates of surgery for benign prostatic hyperplasia. *Medical Care*, 33, 765–70.

Waitzkin, H. (1984). Doctor-patient communication: clinical implications of social science research. *Journal of American Medical Association*, 252, 2441–6.

Wald, N., Chamberlain, J., and Hackshaw, A. (1993). Report of the European Society of Mastology Breast Cancer Screening Evaluation Committee. *The Breast*, **2**, 209–16.

Wald, N., Murphy, P., Major, P., Parkes, C., Townsend, J., and Frost, C. (1995). UKCCCR multicentre randomised controlled trial of one and two view mammography in breast cancer screening. *British Medical Journal*, **311**, 1189–93.

Waldron, J. (ed.) (1990). *Theories of rights*. Oxford University Press, New York.

Ward, S., Heidrich, S., and Wolberg, W. (1989). Factors women take into account when deciding upon type of surgery for breast cancer. *Cancer Nursing*, **12**, 344–51.

Waterworth, S. and Luker, A. (1990). Reluctant collaborators: do patients want to be involved in decisions concerning care? *Journal of Advanced Nursing*, **15**, 971–6.

Watson, M., Greer, S., Blake, S., and Shrapnell, K. (1984). Reaction to a diagnosis of breast cancer. *Cancer*, **53**, 2008–12.

Watson, M., Denton, S., Baum, M., and Greer, S. (1988). Counselling breast cancer patients: a specialist nurse service. *Counselling Psychology Quarterly*, **1**, 23–32.

Watson, M., Murday, V., Lloyd, S., Ponder, B., Averill, D., and Eeles, R. (1995). Genetic testing in breast/ovarian cancer (*BRCA1*) families. *Lancet*, **346**, 8974.

Watson, M., Lloyd, S.M., Eeles, R.A., Ponder, B.A.J., Easton, D.F., Seal, S. *et al.* (1996). Psychosocial impact of testing (by linkage) for the *BRCA1* breast cancer gene: an investigation of two families in the research setting. *Psycho-oncology*, **5**, 233–9.

Webb, P. (1987). Using audio-visual aids for cancer patient education. *Cancer Nursing*, **10** (Suppl. 1), 216–9.

Wei, J.P., Sherry, R.M., Baisden, B.L., Peckel, J., and Lala, G. (1995). Prospective hospital-based survey of attitudes of Southern women toward surgical treatment of breast cancer. *Annals of Surgical Oncology*, **2**, 360–4.

Weihs, K. and Reiss, D. (1996). Family reorganization in response to cancer: a developmenal perspective. In *Cancer and the family* (ed. L. Baider, L. Cooper, and A. Kaplan De-Nour). John Wiley and Sons, New York.

Weiss, S.M., Wengert, P.A., Martinez, E. M., Sewall, W., and Kopp, E. (1996). Patient satisfaction with decision-making for breast cancer therapy. *Annals of Surgical Oncology*, **3**, 285–9.

Wells, R.J. (1986). Informed consent, the great conspiracy. *Nursing Times*, May 21, pp. 22–4.

Wellisch, D.K., Gritz, E.R., Schain, W., Wang, H.J., and Siau, J. (1991). Psychological functioning of daughters of breast cancer patients.

Part I: Daughters and comparison subjects. *Psychosomatics*, **32**, 324–36.

Wellisch, D.K., Gritz, E.R., Schain, W., Wang, H.J., and Siau, J. (1992). Psychological functioning of daughters of breast cancer patients. Part II: Characterizing the distressed daughter of the breast cancer patient. *Psychosomatics*, **33**, 171–9.

Wennberg, J. (1992*a*). We're gradually beginning to democratise the relationship between doctor and the patient. *Medical Economics*, Oct. 5, p. 94.

Wennberg, J. (1992*b*). In *New tools for the informed patient* (ed. J. Willson), p. 33. New Media.

Wennberg, J. (1992*c*). Choose your own treatment (ed. R. Lothman), *American Health*, November.

Whelan, T.J., Levine, M.N., Gafni, A., Lukka, H., Mohide, E.A., Patel, M. *et al.* (1995). Breast irradiation postlumpectomy: development and evaluation of a decision instrument. *Journal of Clinical Oncology*, **13**, 847–53.

White, I., de Matteis, F., Davies, A., Smith, L., Crofton-Sleigh, C., Venitt, S. *et al.* (1992). Genotoxic potential of tamoxifen and analogues in female Fisher 344/n rats, DBA/2 and C57B2/6 mice and in human MCL-5 cells. *Carcinogenesis*, **13**, 2197–203.

White, I., de Matteis, F., Gibbs, A. *et al.* (1995). Species differences in the covalent binding of (C14) tamoxifen to liver microsomes and the forms of cytochrome p450 involved. *Biochemical Pharmacology*, **49**, 1035–42.

Wilkinson, S. (1992). Confusions and challenges. *Nursing Times*, **88**, 24–7.

Wilkinson, S., Maguire, P., and Tait, A. (1988). Life after breast cancer. *Nursing Times*, **84**, 34–7.

Williams, C.J. (ed.) (1992). *Introducing new treatments for cancer, practical, ethical and legal problems.* John Wiley and Sons, London.

Willson. J. (ed.), (1992). *New tools for the informed patient*, p. 33. New Media.

Wilson, R.G., Hart, A., and Dawes, P. (1988). Mastectomy or conservation: the patient's choice. *British Medical Journal*, **297**, 1167–9.

World Medical Association Declaration of Helsinki (1964). Recommendations guiding physicians in biochemical research involving human subjects. Adopted by the 18th World Medical Assembly, Helsinki, Finland June 1964. Amended 29th World Medical Assembly, Tokyo 1975, 35th World Medical Assembly, Venice 1983, and the 41st World Medical Assembly, Hong Kong 1989.

Woolf, S.H. (1997). Shared decision-making: the case for letting patients decide which choice is best. *The Journal of Family Practice*, **45**, 205–8.

Wooster, R., Bignell, G., Lancaster, J., Swift, S., Seal, S., Mangion, J. *et al.* (1995). Identification of a breast cancer gene, *BRCA2*. *Nature*, **378**, 789–91.

Yarnold, J. (1997). Benefits of post-mastectomy radiotherapy. *Lancet*, **350**, 1415–16.

Zigmond, A.S. and Snaith, R.P. (1983). The Hospital Anxiety and Depression Scale. *Acta Psychiatrica Scandinavica*, **67**, 361–70.

Index

Figure and table entries are set in italics. The term 'breast cancer' is implied.